dog owner's

ENCYCLOPEDIA OF

VETERINARY MEDICINE

Illustrations

John Gruen, Scholastics Magazines, Inc. 106, 144, 158

Ernest H. Hart (line drawings) 18, 20, 51-52, 57, 63-65, 71, 73, 82, 112, 134, 160-162

Harry V. Lacey 119

Three Lions (Al Barry 80, George Heyer 48, George Pickow 78, Berni Schoenfield 177)

U. S. Department of Agriculture 35 (drawings) 27, 30, 34

Louise van der Meid 16, 32, 43-45, 54-55, 58-59, 62, 75, 81, 84, 96, 98, 103, 114, 116, 122, 124, 127, 129-130, 135, 138, 142, 150-151, 153, 156, 167-168, 171, 178-179

World Wide Photo 176

dog owner's

ENCYCLOPEDIA

of

VETERINARY
MEDICINE

by

Allan H. Hart, B.V.Sc.

Distributed in the U.S.A. by T.F.H. Publications, Inc., 211 West Sylvania Avenue, P.O. Box 27, Neptune City, N.J. 07753; in England by T.F.H. (Gt. Britain) Ltd., 13 Nutley Lane, Reigate, Surrey; in Canada to the book store and library trade by Clarke, Irwin & Company, Clarwin House, 791 St. Clair Avenue West, Toronto 10, Ontario; in Canada to the pet trade by Rolf C. Hagen Ltd., 3225 Sartelon Street, Montreal 382, Quebec; in Southeast Asia by Y.W. Ong, 9 Lorong 36 Geylang, Singapore 14; in Australia and the south Pacific by Pet Imports Pty. Ltd., P.O. Box 149, Brookvale 2100, N.S.W., Australia. Published by T.F.H. Publications Inc. Ltd., The British Crown Colony of Hong Kong.

" ... and the man strides forward in his
strength, while the woman gives and walks
with inner beauty."

to my wife
Sandy

ISBN 0-87666-287-4

CONTENTS

FOREWORD

Since that eventful day 100,000 years ago, when primitive man and primeval dog first found mutual aid and comfort in their companionship, the dog population has grown gradually ever larger.

New breeds, new concepts of the role the dog must play in its usefulness to man, from hunter, sheepherder, guard, to merely pet and confidante, has broadened and diversified the breed basis enormously. As a necessary result the area of proper and professional care and treatment for the various illnesses to which this vast canine population is heir has had to keep pace with this specie numerical explosion. For today, due to the initial cost of purchase of a well bred dog, the constant monetary outlay for food, barbering, etc., and the rapport that exists between the dog and its owner, the place it has assumed in the family circle, make it imperative that treatment for the dog when it is ill must meet the highest medical standards.

This, we know, has come to pass and today the modern practitioner of veterinary medicine offers, for the care of the animal population, the most advanced medical treatment, techniques and scientific knowledge available.

Dog owners are generally people of vision and intelligence, interested in everything that concerns their animals. They constantly ask "Why?" and "How?", thirsting always for new knowledge that will enable them to give to their pets the best in all areas of canine care and husbandry, and this pertains particularly to the vast areas of canine disease.

Here, then, is the reason for this book—to make available to dog owners a comprehensive treatise on canine diseases, their causes, symptoms, and treatment. The information you find here will perhaps accelerate your recognition of some canine illness and, in turn, give you reason to more quickly seek professional advice or give treatment to your dog, an act that could quite possibly save its life, save you money, and protect you and your family from the emotional stress of the animal's loss.

Hackettstown,
New Jersey

Allan H. Hart, B.V.Sc.

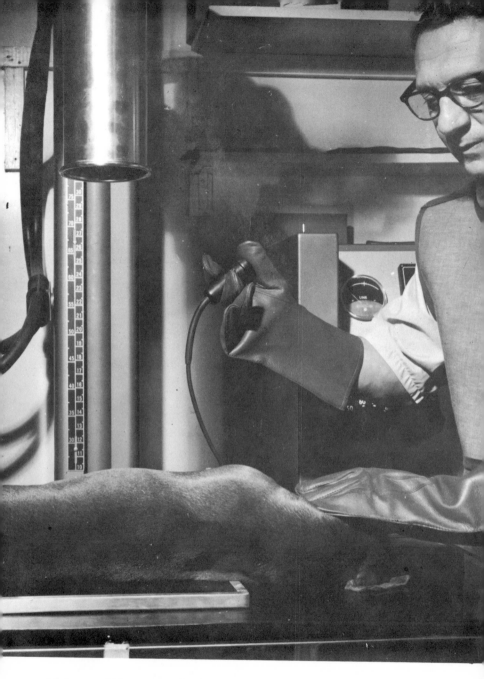

A full range of laboratory services is
performed by today's veterinarian for the benefit
of his clients and the health of his patients.

CHAPTER 1

NUTRITION . . . feeding the dog

Let us first explore the ailments and anomalies that can result from an improper environment, for this is an area over which you, the owner, have control and the power to correct and change.

The most important element in the physical environment which you fashion for your dog is the food or nutrition which you provide to help build the puppy to robust adulthood, or to maintain the adult dog in good health whether the animal is a pet, a working or hunting dog, or a breeding animal.

The animal body must be nourished completely and adequately in all its parts and for all its functions or, like any other engine, it will wear out more quickly than it should, slow down and eventually quit working. Poor feeding practices, lack in nutritional and dietary essentials, will result in deficiencies in many and various sections of the body until the animal's health is so badly affected that it needs medical care and corrective husbandry. In some instances, when undernourishment has been prolonged and drastic, particularly during the time of adolescent growth, the end results can never be completely rectified.

Although the dog is a meat eater by nature, he can utilize efficiently a great variety of cereal and vegetable foods. This ability allows him to retain a nutritional balance in spite of the wide variety of diets we owners impose upon him.

The requirements of dogs vary with breed, size, work and growth. Certainly a Chihuahua and a Great Dane do not have the same growth requirements. The weight of the Great Dane and the huge size he is to achieve, the longer maturing period and the heavier bone growth, make additional nutrition imperative. Just as certainly the maintenance nutritional requirements of a working sled dog in arctic weather greatly surpasses those necessary for a penthouse lap-dog Pomeranian. Unfortunately we do not have room to delve into the requirements of each breed separately, but we will assess the nutritional needs of the average dog.

Common sense and visual results are the best guides to the utilization of this basic information. It is obvious that outdoor dogs need more caloric intake than indoor dogs. Dogs in cold climes need more fats than those in tropical areas, and large boned dogs require higher calcium and Vitamin D in their diets than do toy dogs.

Below are the basic averages found in good dog foods (% per lb. of food).

Nutrient	Dry Dog Food	Canned Dog Food
Moisture	8–10%	70–75%
Protein	13–18.0	4.5–6
Carbohydrate	70	23–25
Fat	5	1.5
Calcium (min.)	1	.4
Phosphorus (min.)	.8	.3
Sodium Chloride (salt)	1.4	.5
Potassium	.8	.3

	mg. per lb. of food		mg. per lb. of food
Iron	22		8
Copper	2.5		1
Cobalt	1.0		0.3
Magnesium	200		70
Manganese	2		.7
Zinc	2		.7
Iodine	.5		.2
Vitamin A	.6		.2
Vitamin D	.003		.001
Vitamin E	20		7.0
Vitamin B$_{12}$	.01		.004
Thiamine	.3	.01	.1
Riboflavin	.8	.3	.3
Pyridoxine	.4		.15
Pantothenic acid	.9		.4

Niacin	4.1	1.5
Choline	560	200

It can be seen that a dog on a canned food diet must consume more food or bulk than one on dry food where the moisture can be regulated. Also, regardless of package amounts, what is important is the availability of the substances for body usage; so often proteins and fats of prepared diets do not do for the dog what the package would have us believe.

Requirements. *Protein* is one of the most important foodstuffs for dogs. Protein requirements for growth, lactation and recovery from debilitating disease, are much higher than maintenance requirements. A 20% good quality protein is necessary for maintenance but 25% is desired for the growing, lactating or recuperating dog. The better quality foods, such as dairy products, are too expensive for inclusion in regular dog foods, so often the food has poorer protein, mostly of plant nature. Heat applied to commercial food for various reasons, further lowers the nutritional value of the protein and/or destroys much of the vitamin content.

The addition of good quality animal protein to a dry food is an excellent procedure. Beef is far better than horse meat as a vehicle of animal protein. Many dogs exhibit digestive disturbances from the intake of horse meat. It also has a higher phosphorus than calcium level. Fish is also a good source of animal protein.

Carbohydrates should not exceed 70% of the diet on the dry basis. They form an important part of the dog's diet although little is known about the exact requirements. Starchy foods, such as potatoes, must be cooked to release nutrient value and prevent the occurrence of diarrhea from the intake of raw starches.

Fat should constitute 12–15% of the dog ration. This is not found in commercial rations because of the possibility of rancidity. Animal fat added with and found in the meat used for higher protein value will help to increase the fat content. Bacon drippings, beef suet and cooking fats are all excellent. Fat requirement increases in the winter and 20% is a good ratio. Too much fat content in the food will cause nausea.

Footnote: Both charts are condensations from "Nutrient Requirements for Dogs," a government publication.

The exact requirements for *vitamins* are often not known. Many vitamins interact and different areas and climates vary requirements. Most commercial foods contain adequate vitamins for the adult dog, but growing puppies (particularly of large breeds), animals recovering from disease, bitches in whelp and lactating bitches, have extra needs that require a good vitamin supplement. The dog requires *minerals* which are present in most foods at maintenance levels. Calcium and phosphorus are the two most important for young puppies (see Rickets). Iron, copper and cobalt are used in hemoglobin (blood pigment) production. It may be necessary to feed iron supplement to dogs that have blood depleting diseases such as hookworm.

Commercially Available Foods

Canned meats are made up of beef and/or horse muscle meat and meat-packing by-products such as lungs, spleen, blood, tripe and bone. These may be artificially colored. Such products are usually a good source of protein.

Canned dog foods of the non-whole meat variety are made of canned meats with the addition of cereals and other plant products. They usually contain so much moisture that many cans of food are needed to supply a dog with proper nutrition. For instance a 50-lb. dog needs $3\frac{1}{2}$ to 4 cans daily while a 50-lb. growing pup needs almost 7 cans. Even then the fat content and many of the other necessary nutrients are on the low side. Canned dog foods of this type are flavorful and tasty but are uneconomical as a complete diet for large dogs.

Biscuits and kibbles are baked-cereal flour products to which meat by-products, milk by-products, yeast, vitamins, mineral supplements, and other vegetable products are added. These, especially the biscuits, contain a high proportion of flour to retain their shape; therefore they are often not well balanced nutritionally. Baking at high temperatures depletes much of the vitamins. These are best used as snacks or fillers and not whole diets.

Dry dog meal and pellets are composed of cereal products such as corn and wheat flakes with fish meal, meat meal, yeast, dry milk solids and other dairy by-products, vegetable by-products, distiller's by-products, vitamins and minerals. These are cooked together and provide a supposedly complete and balanced diet, but owners of large and medium large dogs must realize that most testing has been done on dogs like terriers and Beagles. Molasses is used as a binder for pellets.

In general the best type of basic diet is a mixture of the meal or pellet type foods, with canned meat or whole fresh meat to increase the animal protein and fat. Greater amounts of meat should be used in diets for the puppy, pregnant and lactating bitches, and the dog recovering from a long illness. This mixture should be moistened to form a gruel. Add to this table scraps of meat, cooked vegetable products, fat drippings and gravies. Small amounts of these will not appreciably unbalance the diet and will add variety and flavor. For puppies, lactating and pregnant bitches, and debilitated dogs, vitamin and mineral supplements should be added and, especially for puppies, the whole should be moistened with milk (powdered, whole, or 50% evaporated).

A good weaning diet consists of milk or Esbilac to which hamburger or a similar meat product has been added in small bits. Gradually the solids are increased and puppy or regular dog meals are added. This far surpasses the pablum diets so often recommended by fanciers.

The chart that follows will help the owner to get a general idea of the amounts to feed but these are only an average and dogs, just as do people, vary in the amounts of food necessary to keep in proper condition due to the many involved environmental factors. Remember that, in general, 1 lb. of dry food is equivalent to 4 lbs. of canned food.

Puppies should be fed several times a day. The number of meals and when to reduce them varies with age and breed, but young puppies of 5 or 6 weeks are started on 3 to 4 meals daily. This is cut back to 2 meals at approximately $3\frac{1}{2}$ to 4 months. The puppy will often determine the time. If the puppy will eat three large meals daily without leaving any food and then stay on three meals for the necessary length of time you have nothing to worry about. But if he starts turning up his nose at one or more of the meals or becomes a reluctant eater, then cut back. Sometime between 6 months and a year most dogs are reduced to one meal daily.

Weight of dog	Dry Food (Meal)		Canned Dog Food	
	Adult	*Puppy*	*Adult*	*Puppy*
	lbs. of food	lbs. of food	lbs. of food	lbs. of food
5 lbs.	.2	.4	.55	1.1

10	.34	.68	.93	1.86
15	.42	.84	1.18	2.34
20	.54	1.08	1.52	3.04
30	.78	1.56	2.14	4.26
50	1.25	2.50	3.44	6.90
70	1.75	3.50	4.83	9.68
110	2.75	—	7.60	—

Deficiencies

Vitamin A deficiency causes three possible problems. It causes atrophy of epithelial cells thus predisposing to skin, occular, respiratory and genitourinary disease. It is involved in the activity of bone producing cells. Lastly, the eye pigments needed for vision in dim light are affected, causing night blindness.

The Vitamin D, Calcium, Phosphorus complex is discussed under Rickets in the Pediatric section.

Vitamin E deficiency has been associated with muscular dystrophy in dogs but it probably occurs only under the rarest conditions in nature. Vitamin E has not been shown to be of any value in the fertility of dogs.

Vitamin K deficiency can only occur when bile production is curtailed. The only meaningful problem comes when dicumonal (the active poisonous ingredient in Warfarin) replaces Vitamin K thus causing a blood clotting defect.

Vitamin C is synthesized by the dog so that normally it is not needed. Rare cases of scurvy have been found due to a breakdown in this canine system.

The Vitamin B complex deficiencies are probably second in importance to Vitamin D deficiency as clinical problems. Very briefly we will consider some of the problems.

It might be noted here that while vitamin supplements serve their purpose as general supplements for strict Vitamin B deficiencies, Brewer's yeast, liver extracts and wheat germ are superior to synthetic compounds.

Vitamin B_6 (Pyridoxine) deficiency causes anemia. Replacement via Brewer's yeast is excellent.

Thiamin deficiency causes Chastek paralysis, a paralytic disease characterized by loss of appetite and weight, vomiting, weakness and paralysis leading to death.

Riboflavin deficiency leads to fatty livers and a variable group of problems such as dry skin, muscular weakness, occular changes, anemia and, eventually, sudden death. Liver extracts are the best replacement.

Niacin deficiency will cause blacktongue (pellagra).

Vitamin B_{12} deficiency and Iron deficiency lead directly to anemia.

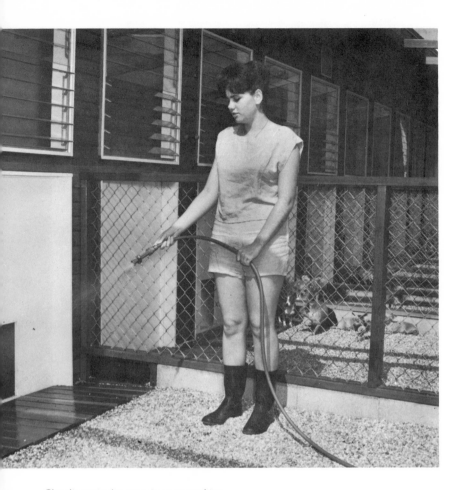

Cleanliness is the most important thing
a lay person can practice to prevent
disease in his kennel. The purchaser should buy
only from a reputable kennel
that is noted for the production
of quality stock, fair prices, integrity,
healthy animals, and kennel cleanliness.

CHAPTER 2

PARASITOLOGY . . . *internal and external parasites*

Worms! Every dog owner has heard of canine worms and most of you have had some practical experience with them sometime during your life as a dog fancier. You will of course get much "practical" advice from neighbors and well-meaning friends. Here, in the introduction to this subject, we hope to dispense with old wives' tales, witches' brews, and folk medicine and give you general knowledge on prevention and control.

Worms do not come from candy! If they did, they would have to have been created spontaneously. The theory of spontaneous generation became outmoded at the time of Darwin. Garlic causes your dog to acquire a very "healthy" breath but it will not act as a worm treatment. Another common idea, that dogs that sleigh-ride their rears along the ground are always infected with worms, is also usually untrue. Roundworms and tapeworms *may* cause this symptom but it is more likely that the dog needs his anal glands emptied. Lastly, tobacco is better smoked in a pipe than used to worm your pet.

Infection can occur in many ways. Worm parasites may enter the body by ingestion, through an insect bite, by penetrating the skin, or via prenatal infection. Infection can be direct or may need an intermediate host. Transport hosts, unnecessary for the parasite's development, can carry the parasite to the dog. Each parasite in its life cycle may use one or more of these methods to continue its existence.

In general dogs with parasitic disease will show signs of unthriftiness, poor hair coat, underdevelopment, diarrhea, vomiting and/or anemia. For the safety of your pet, parasites should be discovered before they become a "disease." You will not find all parasites by examining your dog's bowel movements, some internal parasites are too small, even microscopic. Straining of the stool will sometimes reveal adult worms. But microscopic fecal examination by a trained technician is the only proper and thorough way to a true diagnosis. This method depends upon adult worms being present and producing eggs or larvae. Your veterinarian can perform one of two tests in a matter of minutes for diagnosis. A simple smear of stool will often work, but it is unreliable, especially with those worms which produce smaller numbers of eggs. A much more accurate diagnosis can be made through the flotation method. This entails mixing a small amount of feces in a solution with a specific gravity heavy enough to float the lighter eggs to the top. Using a centrifuge, this can be accomplished in a matter of minutes, or the solution can stand overnight. For the amateur, a super-saturated sugar solution does quite well. Sugar should be added to hot water until it is syrup-like in consistency (specific gravity 1.18 to 1.22). A dip of the fecal mix is taken from the top and placed on a slide for microscopic examination.

From such an examination your veterinarian can select the proper drug to dispense or may require that you leave your dog when harsher or more dangerous treatment is necessary. No one drug can kill all parasites. The average veterinarian has more than a dozen preparations in his pharmacy and correct diagnosis is indicated to enable him to select the drug necessary. The difference between the cost to you in selecting your own preparations from the drug or pet store and your veterinarian's charge cannot pay for the years of experience and training he offers you. If you make the drug selection, you may not be successful and may even kill your dog, from toxicity, or by leaving a lethal worm infection which the drug did not remove.

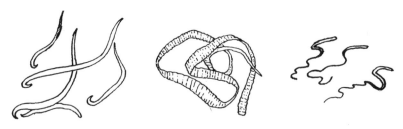

Round worms   Tapeworms   Whipworms

The dog owner plays his most important role in the field of prevention and control. Breaking the link of infection lies in his hands. There are two basic modes of attack;

1. *Eliminating infection in the environment*
2. *Preventing the animal from coming into contact with infected areas.*

Bitches should be checked for parasites and treated before breeding. They should be kept in as clean and new an area as possible. Whelping boxes should be scrubbed, disinfected and even freshly painted. Control of fleas and lice is imperative at all times. Wire bottomed pens are an excellent form of control but are not favored by breeders because they may cause splayed feet. Six month to yearly examinations are necessary on all dogs which have not shown clinical signs. Early detection may be accomplished this way. Dogs showing signs of infestation should be checked upon development of these signs. Dogs being shown, worked in field trials, obedience trials or raced etc., should have more frequent check-ups as they are more apt to come into contact with parasitic infections. Even the house pet may come into frequent contact with infection. Fecal matter left in your yard by infected dogs, flying and crawling insects, and rodents, may bring the infection to your pet. Application of chemicals to dogs runs may help to clean up the premises. Sodium borate applied at 10 lbs. per 100 sq feet of surface will reduce larval inhabitants of the soil. If possible, as the dog is treated and rid of parasitic invaders, the run should be moved.

Nursing treated animals is also an important owner function. Good diet with increased animal protein is an excellent supportive treatment. An increase in vitamins and minerals is also important, especially iron and the vitamin B complex.

Dogs do possess immunity to worms. This may be natural immunity or acquired immunity after infection has been controlled.

External parasites will also be considered here except for those causing specific skin disease which will be taken up in the skin section.

The Public health aspect of the parasites will also be discussed but its purpose is to inform not to frighten the reader. The most common worms of humans are not worms of dogs. The pin worm and the common human tapeworms do not involve your pets. Cross species infection from dog to human is rare but should be understood.

Roundworms

Two species of roundworms, *Toxocara canis* and *Toxascaris leonina*, may infect the small intestine of the dog. The adult worm is slender, white and ranges in size from $1\frac{1}{2}$ to 7 inches long. The life cycle of *Toxocara canis* can be followed in the diagram.

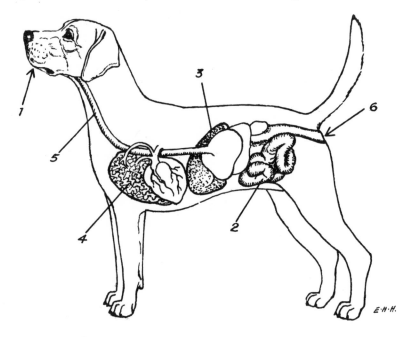

Intestinal round worms (*Toxocara canis*) are
(1) Ingested by dog, usually from food that has come into contact with contaminated ground, or by nursing puppies from the teats of the dam. Prenatal infestation may also occur by larval invasion through the placenta. Each worm egg contains a tiny coiled embryo which is released by the bursting of the shell in the
(2) intestine and then becomes a larva. The larvae pierce the intestinal wall, enter the blood stream, and are carried by way of the
(3) liver to the
(4) lungs. From the lungs they crawl or are coughed up into the
(5) esophagus, to be swallowed and again reach the intestines. Here they lay the eggs which are
(6) voided in the dog's stool. These microscopic eggs generally embryonate within two or three weeks and may remain viable for years.

Aside from this basic life cycle there are intermediate hosts (mice, earthworms or roaches) that can carry the larvae to the dog. Larvae reaching the dog through ingestion of these hosts tend to complete their life cycle without migration to the lungs.

It has also been found that after the adult worm has been eliminated from the dog's system that larvae can encyst in the muscles of the dog. These cause no harm to the pet but in the bitch during pregnancy are activated, probably by hormone changes, and enter the puppy via the bloodstream through the placenta thus causing a prenatal infection. Because of this modification of the life cycle you may find it impossible to raise puppies completely worm free.

Toxascaris leonina has a very simple life cycle as the larvae simply enters the bowel wall to complete development and reenters the intestine after 10 days.

The worm is most dangerous to the puppy and seldom is found in or causes much trouble to dogs over 1 year old. In the puppy three basic effects are found: 1. *unthriftiness* 2. *lung damage* 3. *mechanical interference in the intestine, sometimes to the extent of complete blockage.*

While the wormy puppy is usually pot bellied, he is actually thin along the backbone and ribs. His gums may be anemic. Diarrhea is often present and a dull coat is common. Adult worms are commonly passed in the bowel movement or vomited up.

A variety of medications are available with which to treat your puppy. Many of these, such as n-butyl chloride and tetra-chlorethylene treat more than one worm but are harsh and unnecessary when only round worms are present. Piperazine compounds are very effective, are mild and require no starvation, which is a prerequisite with the others. Treatment usually has to be repeated, often several times, after 10 to 14 days. Dogs treated for round worms as puppies usually build an acquired immunity to the worm at about six months of age.

There are very rare instances where *Toxascaris* has infected man and it is most likely that this was from the ingestion of an intermediate host and not from a puppy.* Again it is quite rare but should be noted. It is caused by ingesting larva which may affect children. General cleanliness and parasite control of your puppy is the watchword to prevent any occurence of this rare disease.

---

*A condition known as *visceral larva migrains* occurs in children. As of 1962 there have been only two cases on record.

Hookworm *Ancylostoma caninum* is the most common species of hookworm found in dogs. Because of the hair-like thinness of the worm and their length ($\frac{3}{8}$ to $\frac{3}{4}''$), they are seldom if ever found by dog owners in the bowel movement. They are a small intestine worm like the the roundworm but are far more dangerous.

They also have a life cycle similar to the roundworm. Besides infection by ingestion, penetration of the skin by larvae and prenatal infection are common.

The hookworm may cause diarrhea and anemia. The condition may become so bad, if not remedied, as to make an animal incompatable with life. A single worm may remove approximately 4 drops of blood per day, therefore, a massive infection of worms can cause circulatory collapse, shock and death.

Once again many drugs can be utilized to eradicate hookworm but most are harsh. A puppy with severe anemia that has to be starved for 12 or more hours for tetracholrethylene or n-butyl chloride may not survive the treatment. A fairly new drug, D.N.P., available only through your veterinarian, is one of the most effective hookworm treatments and is the least toxic. It is injected under the skin without a period of starvation. After treatment, rechecks at 2 to 3 week intervals are necessary to make certain the infection is gone. Bad infections may require 2 or more treatments.

In the area of public health, only four cases have ever been reported of this worm affecting humans as a worm parasite. "Cutaneous larva migrains," can be caused by a species less common than *A. caninum* and is rare in any case.

Whipworm *Trichuris vulpis*, the whipworm, is found in the cecum and upper part of the large intestine of the dog. Three quarters of the total length of the two inch worm is hair-like and the last quarter is about double the thickness. Again they are hard to find unless one strains the bowel movement. The eggs of these helminths take longer to develop so that constant rechecking is necessary to make sure infection after treatment has not recurred. The entire life cycle is spent either in the bowel or the bowel wall and it may take two to three months for the worms to develop into adults.

The female worm lays fewer eggs than most parasites so diagnosis may require careful examination of several specimens. Even then, if your veterinarian suspects the presence of the worm and yet can't find it, he may feel that treatment is rightfully indicated.

The infected dog is unthrifty, may exhibit periodic to constant diarrhea, vomiting, and often a secondary anemia. Blood may be found in the diarrhea, and, if treatment is not undertaken shortly after this, death may occur.

In the past, surgical removal of the cecum or hydrogen-peroxide enemas were used in treatment. Today pthalofyne and newer drugs, milabus and Task, are quite effective. Retreatments and re-examinations are necessary.

Tapeworm Many species of tapeworm may be found in your dog. These can range in size from $\frac{1}{8}''$ to 16 feet in length. The most common types are *Dipylidium caninum* and the *Taenia* species.

Their life cycle differs from the other parasites which we have discussed as they have a compulsory intermediate host in order to complete their life cycle. They occur in one host as a worm and in the other host as a cystic body which parasitizes a specific organ (liver, lung, brain, etc.) depending upon the species of the parasite.

Diplydium caninum uses the flea or louse as an intermediate host and is therefore, very common in dogs. *Taenia* species use rodents, rabbits, sheep and cattle commonly. A dog which catches and eats a rabbit or rodent may become infected. On sheep ranches and cattle holdings, the feeding of raw entrails to dogs will complete the life cycle of the other species.

Echinococcus, the hydatid tapeworm, is not endemic to the United States but is found commonly in Alaska and Canada. This worm is very dangerous to humans as we can be an intermediate host to the cystic form. In countries like New Zealand, where the parasite is endemic, legislation about worming dogs and the feeding of raw entrails has been enacted. Public education is carried out in Australia to combat the problem.

Eggs of the tapeworm are in the body segments and, therefore, are not commonly found in fecal microscopic examination. If you have noticed pieces of "rice-like" bodies in your dog's feces inform your veterinarian when having the dog tested.

Yomesan and drocarbil are commonly used on tapeworms. These require starvation and are harsh on the dog. Most important to the owner is the elimination of the intermediate host as the dog cannot reinfect himself or other dogs.

Heartworm The adult heartworm (*Diroflaria immitis*) can be up to a foot in length. They develop to adult size and inhabit the great veins, the right side of the heart and the pulmonary arteries of the lung.

The female gives birth to microfilaria which invade the blood-stream. Blood samples at this time, examined under the microscope, will show the microfilaria moving between blood cells. The mosquito becomes infected after a blood meal and acts as the intermediate host. In the mosquito they develop to infective larva. After about 2 weeks the mosquito can then infect a new dog. After 3 to 4 months of development in the dog's muscles they migrate to the bloodstream and then to the heart area where, after a second period of 3 to 4 months, they start to produce more microfilaria.

The dog may clinically present a picture of tiring easily, coughing and exhibit heavy, difficult breathing, especially after exercising. In extreme cases the dog may even show all the signs of congestive heart failure.

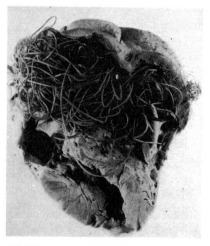

Heart of a dog heavily infested with heartworm. Mosquitoes act as the intermediate hosts for these dangerous worms.

U.S.D.A.

Treatment can be surgical or by drugs. Arsenicals and antimony have been found to be most effective. The adult worms that are killed by the drugs can cause several side reactions; notably fever, cough, and heavy breathing. These may lead to death in 5% or more of the cases treated.

Piperazine compounds are also used but these are primarily for control because they effect only the microfilaria.

Surgical removal must be done by a specialist and is more costly, but the mortality rate is lower.

In endemic areas dogs kenneled outdoors can be treated once or twice a year as a prophylactic measure. Screened runs and pens are an even better preventive measure.

Coccidiosis This parasite is not a worm but a protozoan infecting the intestinal tract. Four species of coccidia have been reported to affect dogs. The disease mainly manifests itself in puppies. Infection is thought to be more wide spread than the clinical picture would indicate.

When the parasite causes disease, which is quite often, it affects an entire litter, usually taking the form of diarrhea, often blood-stained and containing mucous. The puppies lose their appetite and dehydrate quickly. In extreme, untreated cases nasal and occular discharges occur along with coughing. Puppies may die in convulsions. This is not clinically unlike distemper and can well be mistaken for distemper by the layman. Be sure to bring a fecal sample to your veterinarian along with your dog whenever these signs occur.

Several drugs have been recommended for treatment. Sulfona-. mides, wide-range antibiotics and nitrofurazone are most often used. Of these, nitrofurazone is finding most favor. Even with treatment the puppy may not respond and the disease may have to run its course.

When "cured" many dogs become carriers as a state of prem-munity is developed. This is a balance within the dog of parasite and immunity holding all at status quo indefinitely. Bitches which have this state may well pass infection to their puppies. The author experienced this in his own kennel. While other bitches bred during one year showed no infection, in the same environment one bitch (which had had coccidiosis when the author purchased her) whelped and the entire litter became infected with coccidiosis. The bitch herself broke with a bad, new clinical case several weeks after her puppies did. Subsequent litters from other bitches have been clean showing the importance of good sanitation as a preventive measure to keep this parasite from becoming a constant source of trouble in a kennel.

Less Common Parasites

1. An esophageal worm (*Spirocerca lupi*) occurs only with any frequency in the southern states. It definitely occurs, though, more

often than reported. It is not always found and identified as most dogs exhibit no clinical signs. When this parasite causes nodules in the esophagus large enough to be of harm, vomiting or difficulty in swallowing occurs.

The eggs are passed in the feces and diagnosis is made from them. Treatment is unsatisfactory with drugs, and once the nodules in the esophagus are large enough to cause trouble only surgical removal is of help. This condition is rare.

2. Infection with *strongyloides* in the puppy may cause a high mortality rate. This usually affects an entire litter. The puppies can convey the outward appearances of distemper with occular discharges, bloody diarrhea and lack of appetite. Free larvae are found in the bowel movement under microscopic examination. Treatment with dithiazamine iodide is effective only in some dogs. Thiabendazole is very safe and effective. Scientific work with drugs at this time is still experimental.

3. Three parasites affect the lung of the dog as a primary site. Fox lungworm (*Capillaria aerophila*), *Filaroides osleri* (basically the trachea) and the Lung Fluke (*Paragonimus kellicotti*). These are rare and there is no known effective treatment for any of them. They may cause symptoms of respiratory illness but are most importantly involved with secondary pneumonia which may set up in the irritated areas.

4. *Troglotrema salmincala* is a small fluke found in the dog's intestine. It is limited to the west coast and is only important in that it transmits a richettsia which causes salmon poisoning.

5. *Physaloptera* species of worm may be found in the stomach or small intestine. Little is known about them.

6. *The Giant Kidney worm* is also rare but worth mentioning as it is the largest of its type. The female may measure up to 40″ in length. The dog is an abnormal host, this worm being more common in fish-eating wild animals.

7. *Capillaria plica* occurs in the bladder and sometimes the kidney of the dog. It causes no clinical disease and there is no treatment.

8. *A Tongue worm* of ¾″ to 5″ long occurs in dogs. They need an intermediate host and are rare. Treatment is mechanical removal.

Fleas

"*The housing shortage is immense. I can't save enough to give to my true love, a lady flea, a dog on which to live.*" This epic poem was written by my dad many years ago and there is more than just a little humor to be gained from it. Dog owners must strive to keep their pets free of fleas. The dog usually is infected by two species of fleas (*Ctenocephalides canis* and *Ctenocephalides felis*) but may also have human fleas, rat fleas or sticktight fleas. The flea is not host specific. They are wingless insects, the male being smaller than the female.

The flea may carry tapeworm to your dog or act as an intermediate host for heartworm. Heavy infestations may even make an animal anemic. The most common problem arising from fleas is their primary or secondary involvement in "summer" dermatitis. Allergy to flea saliva may even be an initiating cause of this skin trouble. The irritation caused by fleas on already raw skin certainly adds to the condition. It has been shown that with elimination of these pests alone, the skin will greatly improve.

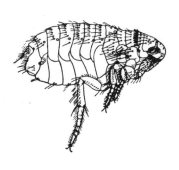 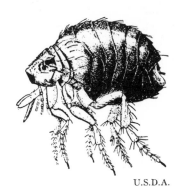

U.S.D.A.

Common dog flea   Sticktight flea

Females lay eggs on the dog and in crevices in the house and furniture. This usually occurs at temperatures of over 65°F. combined with high humidity. One female may lay 500 eggs in her 200 day lifetime. The eggs hatch a larvae form in 2 to 10 days. This form, during its feeding on flea fecal crusts and dried blood may eat the tapeworm eggs of *Dipylidium caninum* and thus become infected. The flea then passes through several stages of larva and pupa which may take anywhere from 3 weeks to a year to produce an adult flea.

Control of fleas is an important owner function. You must clean up the premises as well as the dog. As can be seen from the life cycle, it is not a one time job but must be diligently carried out on a year

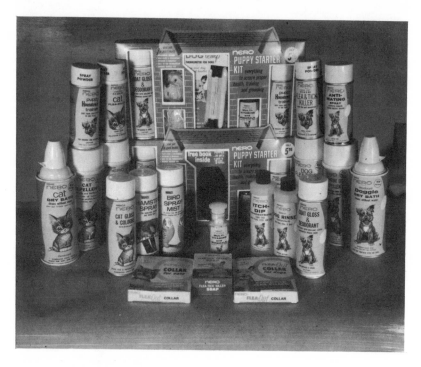

There are a host of cleansers, dips and medications sold in pet shops.

round basis. Many flea sprays, powders and dips have lasting effects for up to 10 days. Sprays which are clean and simple to apply are perhaps the best answer to the problem for the average house pet. Sprays containing 0.5% malathion, 5% DDT, 1% lindane or 3% chlordane are all good and last 5 to 7 days on the dog. Weekly treatment is important. Powders with malathion and rotenone are also good. Rotenone is a quick-kill insecticide and no good on its own for lasting effect. Pyrethrums can be quick-kill or, in newer forms, may have a lasting effect.

Oral medications of organic phosphorus are available but have toxic side reactions on some animals and are expensive.

When infestations are particularly bad, treat the premises as well with a .5% lindane spray or 1% lindane dust. These are toxic to animals, especially cats. Remove pets before treating. Vacuum afterwards and burn the contents.

Remember, for your pet's health, do not increase the recommended amounts or mixtures of dips or sprays thinking they will be more effective; they may just be effective against your pet instead of the fleas. Many of these chemicals store in the animal's fat and need an interval of a week to be metabolized. Treatment carried out too often may eventually build up a toxic quantity of chemical.

Symptoms of toxic poisoning to these chemicals may involve nervous symptoms such as twitching or convulsions. Drooling, constricted pupils and skin irritations, may also be signs of toxicity.

Make sure that the spray or dip you use is fresh. Many sprays are dated. These are the best to buy as you will know when your treatments will become less effective.

So it remains in the reader's hands to make "the housing shortage" too costly for the flea to rent your dog.

Lice

Four species of lice (*Trichodectes felis, Trichodectes canis, Heterodoxus longitarsus, Linognathus setosus*) attack the dog. Three of these are biting lice and one, *Linognathus setosus*, is a sucking louse. These are normally host specific. They are irritating to the dog and the dog's skin, cause anemia, carry tapeworm and cause dermatitis.

When you run your hands through the coat of a heavily infested dog, the coat will feel like it is full of sand.

Treatment is the same as treatment for fleas. Control is easier as the louse cannot live away from the host.

Ticks

Seven types of ticks affect dogs in the United States. Only two of these have wide distribution, the American dog tick and the brown dog tick.

The female is much larger than the male which may be found under her. Blood-engorged female ticks, the size of peas, drop off the dog to deposit several thousand eggs. These hatch within a few months sending out 6-legged larval seed ticks. They seek a host, engorge and drop off and molt into an eight-legged nymph, similar in appearance to the adult. The nymph then finds a host, again feeds and drops off to develop in 10 months into a six-legged adult. The adult finds a new host, mates, and thus completes the cycle. Each stage, nymph, larva and adult, may survive for a year without feeding. Whereas these ticks are three host ticks, the brown dog tick is an exception because it is a one host tick using the same dog for all three feedings. Ticks can infest your house unless care is taken to keep these pests off your dog. Once in the cracks and crevices of your house only a professional exterminator can solve your problem.

If only a few ticks are present on your dog, physical removal may be all that is necessary. I think there are as many home treatments to remove ticks as there are methods for curing hiccups. Simply grasp the tick and with steady traction he will come off. Most let go but you may leave a head behind once in a great while. This is not serious as it will only cause a small pustule at the very worst.

Dips and sprays used for fleas are usually effective (see fleas).

This pest, besides its nuisance value, causes dermatitis and anemia. He may also be a carrier of disease such as canine babesiasis (a protozoan blood infection), or Rocky Mountain spotted fever (a public health hazard in endemic areas). An *Ixodes* species of ticks in Canada can cause paralysis, but removal of the female results in a return to normal. Australia has a similar problem but their *Ixodes* has a toxin which continues to effect the dog after removal. A serum containing antitoxin is necessary for cure or progressive paralysis, finally involving the respiratory muscles, will result in the death of the dog.

The spinose ear tick occurs in the southwestern United States. It causes ear infection (*otitis externa* or ear canker) and may cause hysteria or convulsions. Physical removal and treatment, the same as used to eradicate ear mites, will eliminate this pest.

Myiasis

Myiasis is infestation with fly larvae. The fly will lay eggs in open

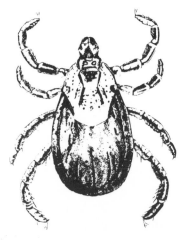
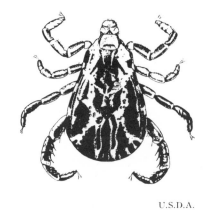

U.S.D.A.

Dog ticks greatly magnified.

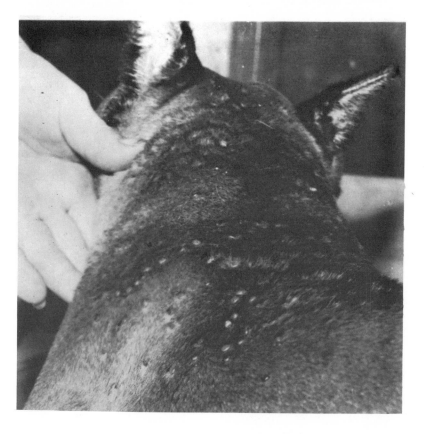

Engorged ticks on a Boxer. These pests
can cause dermatitis, anemia, and
other ills. Insecticides bring quick relief by
controlling ticks and fleas.

wounds, urine stained or fecal saturated hair and skin. The resulting
maggots will then penetrate the skin and cause massive areas of
infection.

Clip away the hair and clean with an antiseptic soap (such as
Phisohex). Flush the area with a dip similar to a flea dip (.03% lindane being excellent). Follow up with antiseptic ointment and a
program of cleanliness.

Control is simple cleanliness. Be particularly careful of fat, long-
haired dogs to be sure that they are kept clean. Clipping a path
under the tail to prevent fecal matter contaminating hair, and urine
staining on bitches, is an excellent method of control.

31

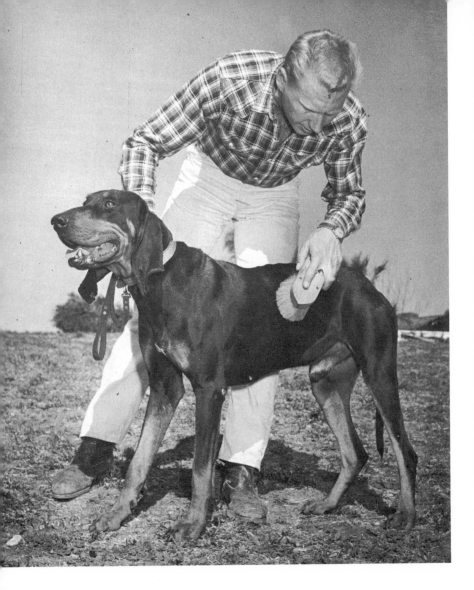

Cleanliness and good grooming help greatly
in the prevention of skin disease.
Also, during the process of grooming,
beginning skin disease, fleas,
and ticks can be seen and quickly treated
and eliminated.

CHAPTER 3

DERMATOLOGY . . . *skin diseases and treatment*

Skin disease is perhaps one of the most frustrating canine conditions to treat. Diagnosis in many cases is difficult. Conditions often tend to recur. Many infections are so totally complicated as to take months of treatment and study to reached finite conclusions and control. Do not become discouraged and go from veterinarian to veterinarian as it will very often only be the very lucky one who correctly diagnoses and finds a cure for a specific condition the first time. A quote from a dermatologist friend sums it all up adequately, "We dermatologists are very lucky. While many of our patients do not get better, they also never die."

Parasitic Skin Diseases

Mange is a household word with dog owners but it is not as common as the uninformed layman believes. Many owners bring their partially bald dog to the veterinarian with the "home diagnosis" of mange.

Mange is caused by mite type *ectoparasites* (external parasites). Two main forms occur in dogs, *Sarcoptic* and *Demodectic* mange.

Sarcoptic mange is caused by *Sarcoptes scabiei*. This mite and its larvae burrow and wander in tunnels in the skin. Their life cycle is about 21 days. They can only survive for a few days when divorced from their natural habitat, the dog. Because of their tunneling, large lesions form which become exaggerated from the dog traumatizing the area. The resulting enlarged lesions make it difficult to find the parasites.

Diagnosis, which is best accomplished by demonstrating the parasite in skin scrapings, may have to be made on clinical signs alone when lesions are widespread and secondary trauma and infection helps the parasite to elude discovery by the laboratory.

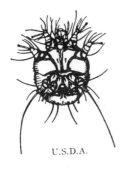

The sarcoptic mange mite, viewed here from the underside, tunnels under the skin causing large lesions. Skin scrapings aid in diagnosis.

U.S.D.A.

The mite prefers the softer skin areas and is usually found on the head, the legs, especially the inside and dorsal portions, and then the body. Hair is lost, the skin becomes thickened, wrinkled and may become covered by an intense puritis. If untreated it may eventually cover the entire body. The dog becomes extremely itchy and scratches incessantly.

Treatment involves the use of an insecticide usually contained in a soothing skin-lotion base. Medicated baths and/or oral insecticides may be adjunctive therapy.

This mite can transfer to the owner and cause scabies. Consult your doctor if your veterinarian diagnoses Sarcoptic mange and you show any itchiness, especially on the arms or other areas with which the dog may make contact. Fortunately it is usually easier to treat you than your pet.

Demodectic mange is caused by *Demodex folliculorum*. This condition has long been known as red mange. It starts with small, dry areas usually on the head or anterior parts of the body and legs. These are traumatized by scratching until red and raw; hence the name red mange. Mites occur in great number, usually making laboratory diagnosis simple and rapid.

This is by far the most difficult parasitic skin condition to treat. In spite of diligent attention by yourself and your veterinarian some cases do not respond. If the condition is fairly widespread the prognosis is poor. Several years ago dogs were destroyed when they had this type of mange. Today's medications certainly control the majority of cases. The mite can also migrate to the lymph nodes, spleen and other organs or lie dormant in hair follicles. These hidden banks of mites may be the reason for unsuccessful treatment.

Long-haired dogs should be clipped and the medication, usually containing insecticides, should be vigorously applied. Medicated baths are good adjunctive treatment for both killing the mite and removing dead skin to make treatment easier. Oral insecticides are often used as adjunctive treatment.

The course of treatment is often several weeks but with small lesions the prognosis is good and the owner should not be discouraged.

Otodectic mange is an ear mite infection and is discussed in the section dealing with ear conditions.

Skin conditions caused by fleas, lice and ticks are common and discussion is included under the parasites heading.

Ringworm

Dermatophytosis, commonly known as ringworm, is a fungal infection of the skin caused by either the *Microsporum* or *Trichoptyton* species of fungus. It is not a worm and is an infection similar in type to "athletes foot" in humans. About 70% of ringworm cases are *Microsporum canis* in dogs. It will fluoresce under ultra-violet light. *Trichophyton mentagrophytes* causes about 10%, while *Microsporum gypsum* causes about 20% of the cases. All three of these fungi are communicable to man and care should be taken in handling the infected dog.

Diagnosis is made by the ultra-violet woods lamp in the case of *M.*

Demodectic mange (red mange) is rather simple to diagnose. Pictured is a moderately severe case. Prognosis is poor if the condition is widespread.

U.S.D.A.

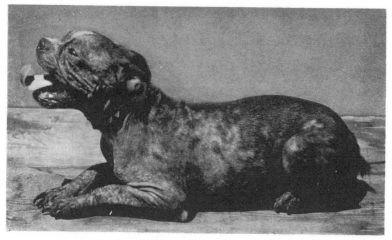

canis while microscopic or culture studies are necessary for positive diagnosis on the others. Sometimes a reasonable diagnosis can be made on the characteristic circular, scaly, bare areas typical of the disease. But often the condition is more generalized making diagnosis difficult without laboratory help.

Oral fungicides, *Griseofluvin,* are very effective. These may be augmented with medicated baths and topical ointment.

Clipping is valuable on long-haired dogs to remove infected hair and allow easier access to the infected areas. Localized treatment may be all that is needed in a few limited cases. Disinfect the area where

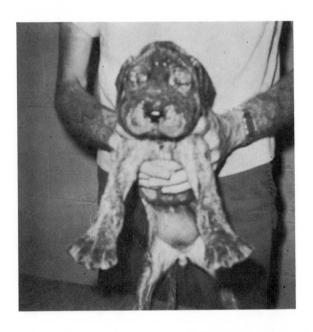

PUPPY ACNE. The use of autogenous vaccines, staphylcoccus-sensitive antibiotics, time, and nursing, eventually changed this six-week-old puppy to a normal Great Dane.

the pet stays and remove old bedding, etc., to prevent transmission to you and reinfection of the dog.

Pyoderma

Pyoderma is a bacterial infection of the skin. Microorganisms invade the skin surface then burrow into the deep layers of the skin. *Staphylococcus* is the most common invader followed by *Streptococcus*

36

corynebacterum and *Proteus*. Superficial infection is common on the abdomen and inner surface of the thighs. It also occurs on the head, lips, nose and between the toes. Puppies frequently get an "acne," usually of the staph type, on their faces.

Deep pyoderma shows a superative infection of the skin and involves skin glands, hair follicles and the deeper layers of the skin.

Superficially infected animals have a good prognosis if proper treatment is given but the condition, even when under expert surveillance, can get out of hand in spite of treatment.

Superficial infections respond well to medicated baths and es-

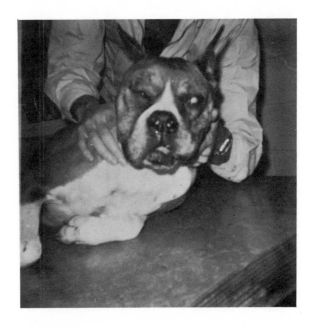

ALLERGIC REACTION. Sensitivity to an insect
bite caused swelling of the face and lips
and the closing of the eye on the right side
of this Boxer's face.

pecially to antiseptic soaps such as Phisohex. Topical lotions or powders with antibiotics are usually applied after bathing. With puppy acne care must be taken to keep the lesions from spreading. Gentle bathing followed by a powder or lotion prescribed by your veterinarian should be used exactly as directed.

Deep pyoderma is much more serious and the prognosis is guarded.

Here the lymph nodes swell, the animal may have ulcers on the skin and deep skin abcesses, with or without fissures to the surface. The patient is often feverish and exhibits anemia and a rise in the protective white blood cells.

These must be treated systematically as well as topically. Abcesses need to be lanced for draining. Hot water baths or soaking may help to break down and drain infection. More often than not the veterinarian must do a culture of the bacteria and a sensitivity test of the various antibiotics to find which is best.

Even with all this intense care and treatment some cases will not respond. Often in these cases a vaccine is made from a culture and the dog is vaccinated by daily doses for several months. X-ray therapy is utilized in very stubborn cases, but this has to be done by a specialist.

In all cases it is important to protect the area of infection from damage by the dog. Tranquilizers, bandages, Elizabethan collars are a few of the methods to be considered.

Allergic Dermatosis

An allergic reaction is a specific reaction of allergen (the agent to which the animal is allergic) with antibodies (agents in the dog which are "anti-allergen") causing histamine release which reacts on blood vessels to cause inflammation.

The animal must have a sensitizing contact with the allergen at an earlier stage. At this time no observable response occurs but a second contact causes a clinical reaction.

Two types of response are seen: The immediate response which manifests itself in minutes, and a delayed response that becomes evident several hours after contact. Parasitic allergies are very common. Dogs become allergic to flea saliva and the result is a very angry dermatitis (see "*Summer Dermatitis*" and "*Fleas*"). The severe, red reaction in *Demodectic* (Red) Mange is an allergic reaction to the mite.

Insect bites may cause hives or severe local swelling. Inhalant and food allergies are becoming more and more recognized in veterinary medicine thanks to scratch tests which are effective in dogs.

These tests, similar to human ones, need more direction toward our dogs for greater use but they do isolate some pollen and dust allergies. They are less reliable on food allergies. Shellfish and eggs are the more common culprits that produce food allergies. Diagnosis depends on trial and error dietary changes.

Drug allergic reactions are the most common. Perhaps the most famous drug reaction is that caused by Penicillin, but any drug can cause skin reactions of varying types. They can sometimes also cause a more general reaction known as an "anaphylactic reaction" which can be fatal.

The second response is the delayed type. This is typified by the tuberculin test where, although no circulating antibodies can be demonstrated, still, after one to three days following contact, a swelling is produced. Contact with simple chemicals to which an animal is allergic can also cause a delayed reaction. Poison Ivy, while typical in humans, has not been proven to be a naturally occurring allergy in dogs, but is a typical example.

Treatment consists of four different attacks.

1. Removal of the source.

2. Drugs which combat the reaction and relieve the dog. *Antihistamines* are specific for allergic reaction but do not relieve all symptoms in some cases. *Corticosteroids* help relieve inflammation and are used as well.

3. Topical therapy of ointments, lotions, a medicated bath are employed when secondary spread from biting and scratching have complicated the condition. Cold applications to insect bites are also helpful when applied immediately after contact.

4. New desensitizing vaccines against specific allergies.

Until you can get your pet to a veterinarian a common antihistamine cold tablet, combined with cold packs, will help to relieve the condition, but these measures will not replace professional care.

Hormonal Skin Condition

Acanthosis Nigricans—This is the commonest and most specific of the hormonal skin complaints. Most of the others are secondarily involved with more serious hormonal disease or physiological imbalance.

Acanthosis nigricans is caused primarily by a thyroid imbalance, but there may be as yet undiscovered modifiers to this disease. It is most common in the Dachshund.

Clinically the dog shows a darkly pigmented hairless skin, especially in the arm pits, then the chest, stomach and hind legs. The skin gets a wrinkled appearance as the condition progresses. The lesions are bilaterally symmetrical. As the condition progresses the skin becomes greasy and scaly. This finally results in a definite odor.

Treatment is based on thyroid stimulation and is often started by a series of injections followed by oral medication. Some cases which have not advanced respond to oral medication alone. *Corticosteroids* offer relief but when they are withdrawn the improvement disappears.

Medicated baths with *antisebboric* shampoos help remove scale and odor and relieve the dog.

Hyperestrogenisen This condition will cause bilateral symmetrical lesions with unbroken smooth skin. In males it is related to Sertoli cell tumor of the testicle. The dogs become "bitchy" in appearance and attract other males. In bitches it usually occurs in virgins over 5 years of age and unspayed. It relates to cystic ovaries with over-active estrogen output.

Surgical treatment in both sexes is desirable. Bitches tend to get *pyometritis* if the uterus is left in and the condition is not rectified. Hormonal treatment with *testosterone* may be helpful with or without surgery.

Occasionally bitches exhibit this condition in late pregnancy or when nursing puppies. It is probably basically both hormonal and nutritional. The condition is usually self-rectifying after the pregnancy and nursing time ceases.

Adrenal hyperfunction results from a hypertrophic adrenal gland or from excessive stimulation from the pituitary gland due usually to tumors (the pituitary gland is a main control gland to many endocrine glands and is located in the brain area).

Hair loss is usually on the flank and flecky over the rest of the body. The stomach is often soft and pendulous.

Hypopitutarism is also usually caused by pituitary tumor. The dog is obese and has a soft fuzz over the body instead of hair. Diabetes insipitus may complicate the condition.

Hypergonadism causes hair loss on the tail and thigh and increased urination.

Seborrea is a dermatosis caused by the increased activity of sebaceous glands locally or over the total body.

Behind the ears, on the face, the neck, the shoulder and base of the tail are the commonest areas. The skin becomes scaly and greasy crusts surround the bases of the thinning hairs. Itching is not usually too severe but the dog is quite odorous.

Unsaturated fatty acids and vitamins A, B complex and D, tend to help. *Corticosteroids* and *estrogens* are often used supportively. Arsenic injections have also been applied. External bathing with cold tar soaps helps not only the skin but also removes the offensive odor.

Summer Dermatitis (*Also called summer eczema, and seasonal dermatitis*)

This condition is most prevalent during the summer months.

Once afflicted the dog becomes susceptible to recurrences. Each year the condition may start earlier in the spring and last late into the fall or may become so chronic as to be year round.

It usually starts fairly suddenly and spreads rapidly. The most common area is along the rump and back area. The area is raw and inflamed. The animal scratches incessantly and further traumatizes the area. The lesions may become infected with bacteria or other contaminants until the affliction is truly a "mixed-bag" of skin ills.

What causes it is still a great question. Obviously many things are involved, and I feel it is a syndrome rather than a single disease. Various veterinarians have various theories about the prime cause but no one explanation fits all cases.

A. Predisposed by hot and humid weather
B. Factors blamed as prime causes
    1. Fleas
    2. Food allergies
    3. Grass fungus
    4. High energy or fatty foods
    5. Poison Ivy
    6. Bacterial infection
    7. Other allergies
    8. Sunburn
C. Factors causing complications
    1. Self-trauma
    2. Secondary infections
    3. Infections with other skin conditions

First we must examine section B. Many of these causes are imaginary, have no scientific basis, or are outmoded, but I have heard all of them used as a previous diagnosis when treating an old or referred case. I do not know what causes it but I do know that fleas may be one of the major causes and they certainly will make this type of skin disease worse. No food allergies, grass fungi nor poison ivy have ever been proven to be a true cause. No doubt some foods and other allergic conditions can become involved and may be primary or secondary. Bacterial infection often becomes involved secondarily but could be primary. These conditions are frequently disguised by a recognizable specific skin condition. This could be primary in many cases before self-mutilation makes the condition almost unrecognizable.

Treatment is directed at three areas.

1. *Stop self-mutilation.*
2. *Find and treat the underlying cause.*
3. *Treat the infected area for relief and healing.*

Self-mutilation is usually treated with *corticosteroids* to reduce the itch. Many of the preparations contain a mixture directed at skin improvement. Sometimes topical ointments with local anesthesia stop itching. Dressings may be employed.

Identification of the underlying cause will not be easily forthcoming. Until some of the symptoms are relieved and control is gained it may not become apparent. But when it does, specific treatment is applied.

Lotions, ointment, powders and medicated baths, will all help heal the skin. Antibiotics may be necessary where bacterial invasion has occurred. Flea control is imperative. Where it is obvious that fleas are the primary cause it may be found that the dog has become allergic to the flea saliva so that one flea can do the damage of an army of fleas to that specific individual. Flea antigen injections and careful flea control is often employed.

Summer Hot Spots (*moist eczema*)

These are rapidly appearing areas of moist infection. They are most common in the summer and are usually bacterially infected. They appear very suddenly and may spread rapidly in a few hours. Different parts of the body are infected. They are very itchy and the dog tends to damage the area. The dog may vomit, run a temperature and the regional lymph nodes may become enlarged. The lesion is usually moist and yellowish in color. These respond very well to topical ointments containing anti-inflammatory drugs, antibiotics and soothing emollients. Systemic anti-inflammatory and antibiotic treatment is often used. The area should first be clipped and cleaned well. Antiseptic soaps are sometimes used to remove debris and dirt.

General cleanliness and grooming helps to prevent hot spots as they are more common on dirty, ungroomed dogs.

Lick Granuloma

This is a chronic *granulomatous* dermatitis (a raised, thickened, lesion) and occurs mainly on the dorsal surface of the pastern area. No one knows why the dog licks the area but unless professional advice is sought these may become "incurable." Small ones respond to local injections of corticosteroids but larger ones can return after all local treatment and surgery have been exhausted. X-ray therapy by a radiological specialist is the treatment which may bring about a cure.

Nasal Solar Dermatitis

Commonly called "Collie nose," is almost always limited to Collies, Shetland Sheepdogs and their crosses. The apparent cause is a photosensitivity to sunlight. The nasal area and along the muzzle

Collies, Shelties, and crosses of these breeds are candidates for nasal solar dermititis, commonly called "Collie nose." The cause seems to be hypersensitivity to sunlight.

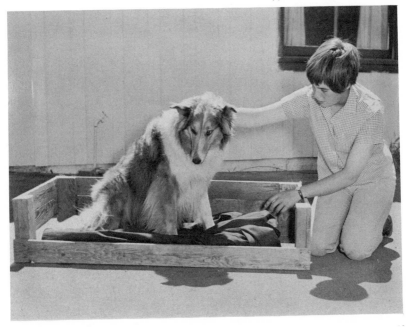

regresses during the winter and usually becomes worse with each passing year.

Ointments and painting with black marking pencil gives some help preventatively but only temporarily. Tattooing is a very helpful treatment. It helps to prevent and cure but it should be undertaken early before years of exposure have made the condition extensive.

Interdigital Cysts

Commonly occur between the toes. They have a tendency to recur after treatment. The attending veterinarian may lance and cleanse the area, he may cauterize, he may completely remove them surgically or treat them medically.

Interdigital Granulomas

Two types occur; the Pyoderma or the foreign body type. Awns, ingrown hair, sticks, are some of the foreign bodies that cause it. Often the area must be lanced and the foreign body removed. Heat, soaking and antibiotic ointments are routine treatment.

Rhabditic Dermatitis

A rare, acute dermatitis of dogs caused by a worm parasite. *Rhabditis strongyloides*, invading the skin. This is a saprophyte

Hyperkeratosis, or horny growths, is a rare condition affecting the pads of the feet, especially of Cockers and Irish Terriers.

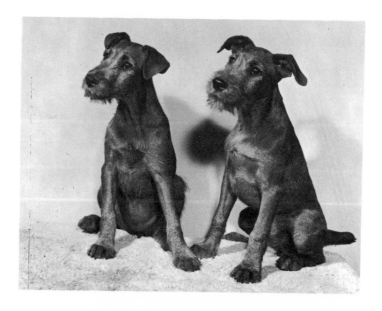

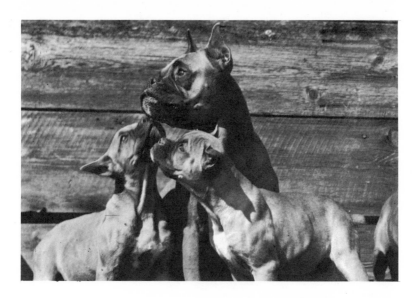

There are several varieties of malignant skin tumors, and they can occur anywhere on the skin. One of these malignancies is a mast cell carcinoma which is commonly associated with Boxers.

usually found in soil in decaying matter. Worms are found in skin scrapings made from pustules formed in the skin.

Control and cure is expected with improved hygiene.

Tumors

Many kinds of tumors develop in the skin. About 80% of skin tumors are benign. The incidence of these increases with the onset of middle age.

Warts are very common especially in older dogs and are not dangerous.

Fatty tumors also occur with some regularity in older dogs. These are often large but are usually benign.

Horny growths (*Hyperkeratosis*) occur on the pads especially among Cocker Spaniels and Irish Terriers. This rare condition has a hereditary base. Treatment consists of soaking and trimming off the growth when it interferes with walking.

Perianal adenoma is a benign growth under hormonal influence occurring around the anus. They ulcerate and hemorrhage easily. The condition appears commonly in old Cocker Spaniels. Surgical removal or cauterization with castration is often done.

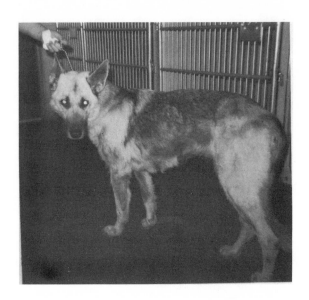

A hormonal skin condition. It was controlled in this instance by spaying and the use of male hormone.

Excessive amount of "elephant skin," caused by constant contact of the elbow with hard surfaces.

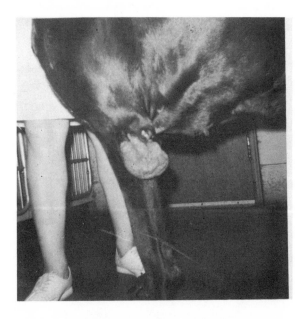

Fibroma, a benign tumor made up of basically fibrous connective tissue cells, is commonly found in the dermis (skin).

Sarcomas, carcinomas, malignant epithelioma and *adenocarcinoma* are the common malignant skin tumors. They can occur anywhere in the skin. *Adenocarcinoma* commonly involves the skin glands. Mast cell sarcomas are commonest in Bostons and Boxers. *Squamous cell carcinoma* is probably the most common *carcinoma*. Removal of the malignant type is often impossible as the skin invasion can be very extensive. However, it should be tried and should be quite radical taking as much tissue in the "healthy" area as possible. The regional lymph nodes are often taken to see if the tumor is spreading. Histopathological studies should be done more frequently than is common, but often cost and available facilities discourage this procedure. X-rays of the chest are necessary wherever malignancy is spreading as the lungs are a prime secondary target. X-ray therapy is also useful and may slow growth and prolong life. The prognosis is always guarded, and poor in reference to malignant tumors.

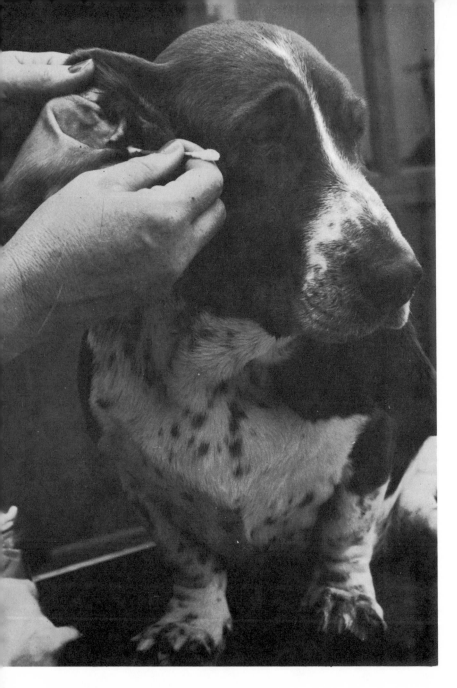

Keeping your dog's ears clean is important. If
they are persistently dirty or odoriferous you may
be dealing with canker. Consult your veterinarian.

CHAPTER 4

EYES AND EARS...*diseases and treatment*

The eyes and ears of your dog are vulnerable areas, a prime target of the elements, of the vagaries of wind and rain and weather, of odd bits and pieces of matter, sometimes microscopic, that can cause injury or irritation.

The dog's eyes and ears are close to the ground and he does not possess prehensile hands that can aid him in brushing or cleaning away dangerous debris that might collect in these vital areas.

Added to these obvious exterior sources of irritation are the many anomalies of various kinds, including those of a glandular, congenital and/or hereditary base that can affect these very important sensory agents of the dog.

The Eye

The dog owner should recognize changes in his dog's eyes and without delay seek veterinary advice. Examine the eye for increased redness, discharge, dullness, opacity, or foreign bodies. Note changes in the size of the eye or the size of the iris opening. Under light the iris is more closed, making a small pupil, and in the dark the pupil is wide. Watch for uncontrolled movements of the eye such as the eye moving sidewise and snapping back in a regular pattern. A problem in one eye is usually a localized problem while an anomaly of both eyes usually heralds a generalized body condition. Conditions affecting the nervous system can also cause ocular changes.

Inflammations

Conjunctivitis is an inflammation of the mucus membranes lining the eyelids and reflected on to the eyeball.

There can be a rather clear discharge to a purulent discharge.

Conjunctivitis accompanies respiratory infections especially the respiratory form of distemper. It is commonly found in chronic disease where the animal is generally run down: e.g. parasitic infestations. It can be caused mechanically by dust, wind, straw, foreign bodies, *entropian* (turning in of edge of eye) and *ectropian* (turning out of edge of eyelid as in the Bloodhound). Dogs who ride with their heads out of the car window commonly suffer from this complaint. It is a common problem in "pop eyed" breeds where the dog has blocked tear ducts and becomes less resistant to infection. Also those dogs with a lack of pigmentation around the lids or the edge of the nictating membrane are more susceptible. Allergies, snow or ultraviolet light, can also be causative agents. Or the inflammation may simply be due to a localized bacterial infection.

Treatment is carried out by eye drops or ointments often containing substances to relieve pain or itch, but if the conjunctivitis is only a reflection of a general body condition it is essential that this condition be identified and treated as a primary target.

Keratitis

Keratitis is an inflammation of the cornea of the eye. The cornea is made up of five layers. The fourth layer, Desemet's membrane, is a stringy elastic layer that often remains intact when the other layers have degenerated.

Keratitis will produce *vascularization* (increase and growth of area blood vessels), engorgement of normal vessels, loss of transparency, ulceration or cellular or pus invasion of the aqueous humor behind the cornea.

This kind of inflammation may be caused by injury or infection. *Pannus* is a specific type of connective tissue infiltration, the cause of which is unknown. It usually occurs in both eyes and is seen most often in the German Shepherd. It produces a film which eventually covers the entire cornea and results in blindness.

Ulcers are common and usually the result of injury. They are seen in litters of pups where nails are not trimmed and the puppies scrap a lot. They are also common in pop-eyed toy breeds where eye protection is not as good as in other breeds. Ulcers vary in importance and type as to the number of layers involved. Cauterization or surgical repair is often necessary to gain healing. Pigmented cells may invade the cornea as a result of *keratitis.*

Treatment for most *keratitis* conditions utilizes ophthalmic ointments with antibiotic and anti-inflammatory drugs. Heat packs are often of great help for home nursing after your veterinarian has prescribed.

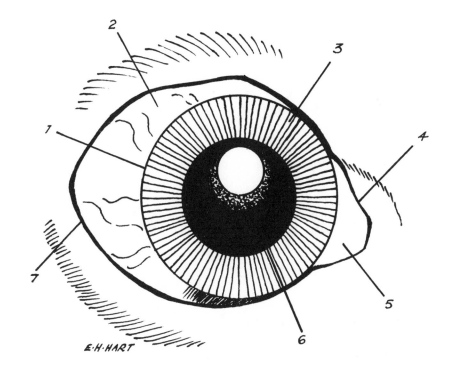

E·H·HART

VISIBLE PARTS OF THE CANINE EYE

1. Limbus   2. Sclera   3. Iris
4. Medial canthus   5. Membrane nicitans
6. Pupil   7. Lateral canthus

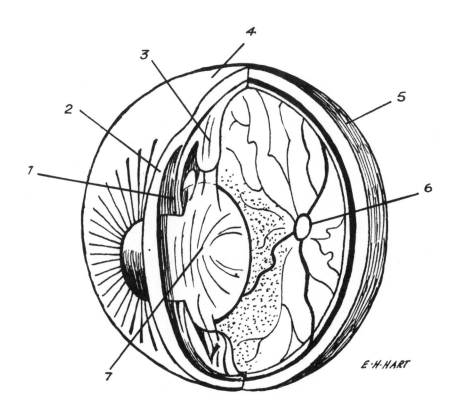

CUTAWAY OF CANINE EYE

1. Iris   2. Cornea   3. Ciliary body
4. Sclera   5. Choroid
6. Optic disk   7. Lens

Ulcers usually are treated with antibiotic ointment and hot packs 3 or 4 times daily. Atropine is often employed. Surgery eventually may be indicated.

Uveitis

Uveitis is inflammation of the uveal tract (may involve the iris, ciliary body and choroid, individually or in combination). It can be an extension infection from deep *keratitis* or may result as secondary to any focal infection or to many diseases.

Glaucoma

Glaucoma is increased intraocular pressure usually from the inability to remove excess fluid (aqueous humor). The eye looks enlarged and swollen. The cause of primary *glaucoma* is unknown, but secondary *glaucoma* results from an abnormality inside the eye such as a dislocated lens or intraocular hemorrhage. Retinal degeneration may occur resulting in blindness.

Glaucoma is usually treated with *miotics* (drugs which cause contraction of the pupil). These drugs are often not tolerated by the dog causing diarrhea, vomiting and other toxic reactions. Listen carefully to your veterinarian and do not overuse the drug. Sometimes surgical intervention can open new avenues of drainage.

Cataract

Cataract is an opacity of the lens. It continues to destroy the lens until blindness results. Usually when owners recognize the condition the *cataracts* are mature and have already interfered with sight.

Cataracts are basically of two types; those in the aged dog, which are the commonest, and juvenile congenital cataracts.

Treatment usually consists of surgical removal of the lens. This, if complications do not set in, will result in a return of sight to the pet. He may not be able to read a newspaper afterward because of an inability to change focus, but if he was able to read one before I would consider him worthy of special eyeglasses.

Retinal Disease

Congenital or hereditary *retinopathies* are caused by degeneration, detachment, abnormal development, or tumors. Bedlington Terriers have hereditary detachment while Irish Setter puppies are predisposed to retinal atrophy. The Collie eye can also be considered the result of an abnormal retinal development. These same problems can arise unrelated to heredity but as yet the cause or causes are unknown. Treatment is, as yet, unsuccessful.

Trauma to the retina is uncommon but can occur. The result can be hemorrhage or detachment. Treatment here may be very successful.

Most retinopathies are secondary to general systemic disease such as; distemper, coccidioidomycosis, septicemia, and nutritional deficiency (especially Vitamin A), all common causes.

Harderian gland

The gland of Harder is located under the third eyelid. The gland may swell and protrude over the edge of the eye causing irritation and *conjunctivitis*. Boston Terriers and Cocker Spaniels are among the breeds more commonly afflicted. Surgical removal is the simple and recommended treatment.

Lacrimal Apparatus

The *Lacrimal apparatus* consists of the gland which secretes tears and the duct which carries them away.

Administration of eye drops.

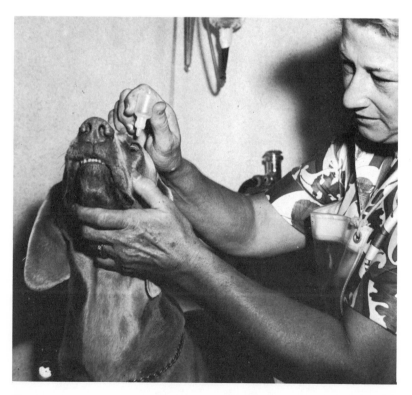

The gland may become inflamed from extension infection due to *conjunctivitis* or may fail to secrete enough fluid, resulting in dry, irritated eyes. The duct may be congenitally absent or malpositioned. Surgical corrective measures to open the duct may be attempted.

Collie eye, entropian and ectropian, is discussed in the chapter on pediatrics.

The Ears

Under normal conditions your dog's ears should be clean other than for external dirt which may contaminate the external ear canal and the ear flap. Oils such as mineral oil are excellent for cleaning. Insert a few drops of oil and gently massage the ear. Remove the debris with cotton or cotton swabs. It is difficult to injure the ear drum if normal care is taken as the ear makes an almost right angle turn going down from the external surface and then inward to the eardrum.

Administration of eye ointment.

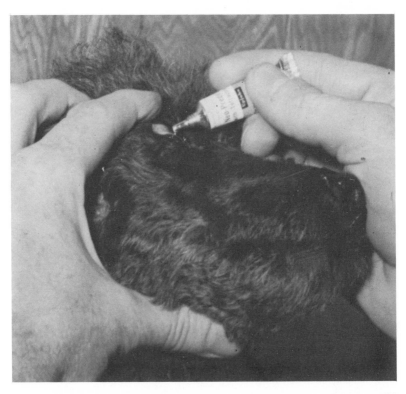

Certain breeds and types of dogs are more prone to various infections of the ear. Flap eared dogs are more likely to develop ear canker and haematoma simply because of their anatomy. The ear flap covers the ear allowing infection to cook up inside like a pot with a cover on it. Unlike most other breeds, the Poodle grows hair in the ear which, unless removed, can predispose this breed to ear infection.

Otitis Externa (Ear Canker)

The cankered ear is swollen and very sensitive. There is discharge varying in amount and type depending on how long the condition has existed and what type of agents have invaded it. At the start the discharge is watery and discolored. It often becomes tarry and black showing the presence of blood. Soon it turns purulent, and odorous, and the surface of the canal may break and ulcerate. As the condition progresses into a chronic stage granulation tissue forms and the ear becomes "cauliflowered" to the point of closing the ear canal, which results in impaired hearing.

If the condition is caught early it responds very nicely to medical treatment, usually clearing up within a week's time. But, if allowed to reach a chronic stage, treatment is lengthy and often best left entirely in the veterinarian's practiced hands. He will often hospitalize the animal in order to give sedatives to allow a complete irrigation of the ear. Continuous treatments with local mixtures of antibiotic and antifungal medications are used. Systemic treatment is helpful in very bad cases. If proliferation has started, or the condition is not resolved medically, then surgical treatment is necessary. With surgical treatment the first part of the ear canal is removed so that the right angle is gone and a straight ear canal remains.

This removes the vehicle that stews the infections, by-passes the proliferated area and allows good drainage.

Otitis Media

Otitis media is an infection of the middle ear. It is usually secondary to *Otitis Externa* or may enter via the eustachian tube. Less common is primary infection in the middle ear.

Primary otitis media show no discharges but the animal shows pain in the base of the ear and may show incoordination and a tilting of the head. The animal is also depressed and off its food.

Secondary infections usually show discharge extending from the middle ear to the external ear.

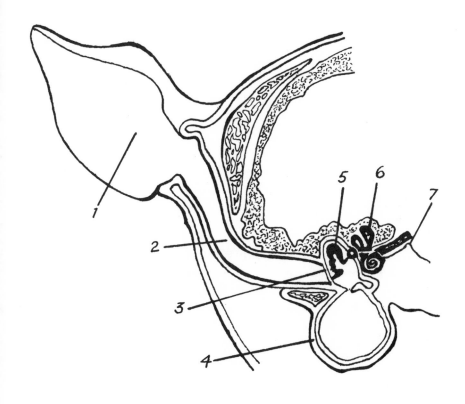

CUTAWAY OF CANINE EAR

1. Pinna 2. External canal 3. Tympanic membrane
4. Tympanic bulla 5. Ossicles
6. Bone labyrinth 7. Otic nerve

Primary cases respond well to systemic antibiotic treatment. Surgical intervention is sometimes necessary.

Secondary cases are treated systemically and locally but surgical intervention is often also necessary.

Ear Mites (*Ear Mange*)

Ear infection often results from the invasion of *Otodectic cynotis*, the ear mite. The animal shakes his head and scratches at the ear. The discharge is usually black and tarry from blood. Secondary ear canker is common in long standing cases.

The mite can usually be seen under the microscope. It is related to the mites that cause skin mange.

Examination of ears may reveal ear canker or ear mite infection. Early diagnosis by your veterinarian is desirable and immediate treatment necessary to prevent deep-seated trouble.

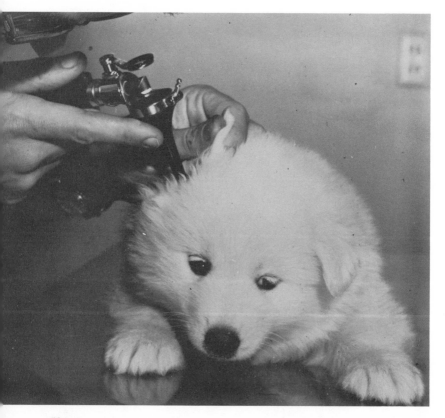

Treatment should be carried out for 10 to 14 days in order to kill new broods of mites which are hatched during treatment. Keep the ear clear (see "cleaning ear," under *Otitis Externa*). In very bad cases external parasite control with powders and sprays will get those mites not in the ear canal. Also, in bad cases, weekly treatment may be advisable for several weeks after apparent cure.

Medications used for mite infections contain an insecticide with or without antibiotics. Be careful to use only as your veterinarian advises as many of the medications can injure the ear if used too frequently.

Ear Haematoma

A *haematoma* is a large blood pocket most commonly seen in the ear flap. It is produced by trauma causing a rupture of small vessels and the formation of a large fluctuating swelling in the ear flap. It is a common secondary complication to ear mites and canker due to the constant scratching and shaking of the ear. It usually involves only the concave surface of the ear. Unless attended to, the untreated course of healing will commonly result in a crumpled and cauli-flowered ear.

Treatment by asperation may be successful on small haematomas, but usually surgical intervention is necessary.

Deafness

Congenital or inherited deafness is not uncommon. Bull Terriers, Scottish Terriers, Sealyham Terriers, Fox Terriers, Border Collies and Dalmatians are most commonly predisposed as breeds. In blue merle Collies there have been reported ear abnormalities and deafness. It is therefore most common in predominantly white and "harlequin-like" colors. Geneticists tell us that a doubling of the harlequin gene will produce deafness.

Deafness is sometimes hard to identify in active puppies. It is necessary to watch the dog for unusual behavior. Non-cocking of the ears, altered voice and less barking than normal are signs of deafness. Test the dog, when his is not looking, with hand clapping, shouting and whistles. Remember stamping the feet or slamming a door produce vibrations which the dog can feel and therefore respond to.

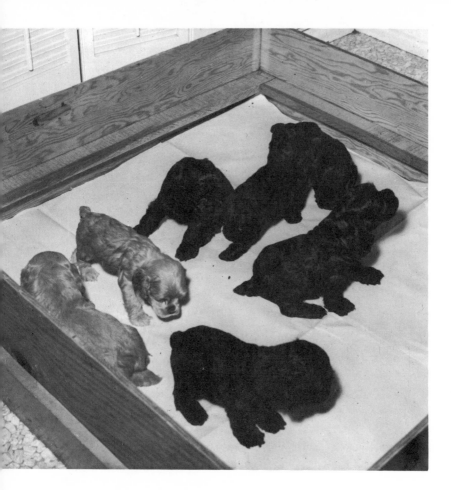

Use the proper whelping box and give the bitch
good care before and after whelping.
Watch mother and puppies closely and at the
first sign of trouble contact your veterinarian.
Quick attention can save the lives of pups and
sometimes the dam if illness strikes.

CHAPTER 5

PEDIATRICS...puppy diseases and treatment

Fortunately for most dog owners "mamma" has an instinctive, built-in drive to care for her puppies. Occasionally a nervous bitch with her first litter will become confused and may have to be helped. As experience with past births accumulates the bitch becomes more and more able to care for her pups and will even help you to wean them.

Keep the bitch in a dry environment with a temperature of approximately 75 degrees; she will in turn supply her body heat to keep the puppies in even warmer surroundings within the whelping box.

Safe whelping boxes can be made by utilizing "nesting" straw so that the puppies will roll from corners to the center, or by building your whelping box in rectangular form with a "puppy lip" around the inside so that the bitch cannot crush a puppy against the sides of the box.

I prefer the latter pup pen. The box is simply lined with newspaper which is easy to change and can be kept much cleaner, with less dust and less danger of sharp, poking sticks. The box should be of a size to fit your breed. Too large and the pups may crawl too far away from the mother–too small and the bitch may have trouble finding room and may sit on the puppies. Extension sides can be added to turn the box into a pen after the puppies are weaned.

Weaning

Weaning time depends upon many factors – the condition of the puppies, the condition of the bitch, the amount of mother's milk available, and the breed. Probably optimum weaning time is from 5–6 weeks of age, but if the bitch was in poor condition and is further run down from her pregnancy, whelping and feeding the whelps, the puppies can be weaned as early as 3 to 3½ weeks. Supplementary feeding and nursing is a good idea after the puppies are 3 weeks of age if the bitch is starting to show the strain. The amount of supplementary feeding and nursing depends upon the condition of the bitch.

If the puppies are not doing well on the bitch, supplementary feeding by tube or bottle (see orphan pups) is excellent. Usually this is necessary when the bitch is low in milk or has a large litter. Lack of milk in a bitch is always a good reason for early weaning. Large breeds, such as the German Shepherds and Great Danes, seem to wean early and do well. One of my clients, a long experienced breeder of top Great Danes, tends to wean between 3–4 weeks of age and has never encountered a nutritional problem.

Puppies should be weaned on basically a milk diet. This can be ordinary evaporated milk (preferably used over whole milk as it is closer to the bitch's natural milk), but if economics allow, or if the puppy's stomach is sensitive to cow's milk, Esbilac, Vetalac (both

Supplementary feeding by tube or bottle (as in illustration) is necessary if it is found that the puppies are not doing well on the dam.

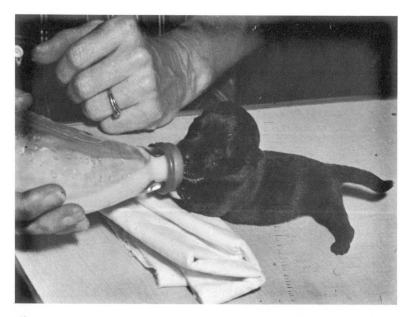

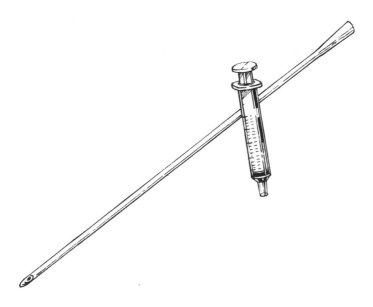

These are the tools necessary for feeding the orphan puppy (or for supplementary feeding). Illustrated are a number 8 to 10 French catheter, and a 10 to 30 c.c. hypodermic syringe.

bitch's replacement milks) or goat's milk can be used. Cow's milk is actually higher in lactose content than is desirable. The addition of egg yolk and albumin to cow's or goat's milk, or evaporated milk, will help to improve it in the right direction. Gradually add whole ground meat to the diet and then, after a few days, a good puppy food. The puppy foods, now made by several companies are far superior to pablum or human cereals. They should be made into a sloppy gruel for your puppies. Feed them a minimum of three times daily, preferably four times when first weaned, and up to 6 times daily if weaned early.

Orphan Puppies

It the bitch dies, or is unable to care for her puppies from birth, you must take over the job. This is a challenging task but not nearly as difficult as it may seem.

Feeding should be done up to 6 times daily and through the night. But feeding every 8 hours has proven successful and you should have at least some time-break at night for yourself. Use a small doll's bottle with a soft nipple or a specially supplied puppy nurser. Even easier for you, and perfectly alright for the puppy, is feeding by stomach tube. A French catheter #8–10 can be supplied by your veterinarian or drug store. Measure the tube length from mouth to stomach (just at the last rib is approximately right), then moisten the tube, gently force the puppy's mouth open and pass the tube over the tongue and slowly into the throat. With steady pressure the puppy will begin to swallow the tube. When you reach the mark you formerly made, you are there. Attach a syringe, preferably one marked in millimeters, and squirt the milk down the tube. Remove the tube. Once you are proficient in this method you can feed an average litter of 7 puppies in approximately 20 minutes. In breeds the size of Beagles, 5–6 cc. per feeding on a 4 feeding per day basis is usually enough to start with, while with Bassets 8–10 cc. may be needed. Increase and judge the increase by the size of the puppys' stomachs.

Feeding the orphan puppy through the use of stomach tubing requires a number 8 to 10 French catheter and a 10 to 30 c.c. hypodermic syringe. It may be necessary to increase the size of the tube as puppies of large breeds grow.

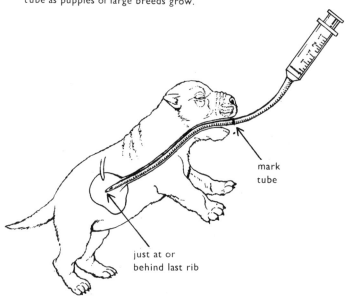

mark
tube

just at or
behind last rib

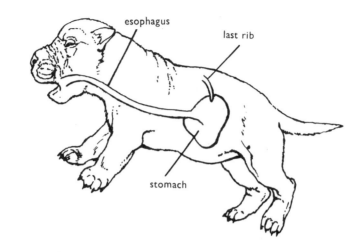

esophagus

last rib

stomach

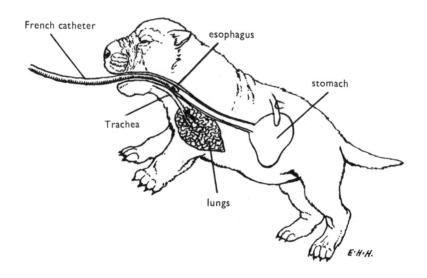

French catheter

esophagus

stomach

Trachea

lungs

E·H·H·

Trachea is too small to allow a number
8 French catheter to pass
unless puppy is over
ten days old.

Obviously every puppy in a litter is of different size and the amount should vary slightly. The stomach should be round and full-appearing without being hard. Overfeeding will cause immediate regurgitation and the puppy should be held head down and the milk cleared from nose and mouth so none is breathed into the lungs. Reduce the amount of milk when this happens.

It is almost impossible to pass the tube into the lungs when the puppies are just born but as the puppies grow, particularly in larger breeds, it is often necessary to replace the tube with a larger one.

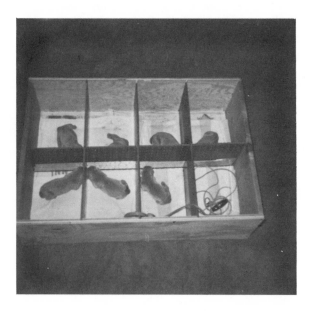

An elaborate but successful incubator that has proved quite effective in raising orphaned puppies.

A better way of measuring the needs of the puppy is through mathematics.

Puppies require 60 calories per pound per day when in an incubator and 100 calories per pound per day if not. Formulas are approximately 1 calorie per cc. Therefore a $\frac{1}{2}$ pound puppy in an incubator needs about 30 cc. of formula per day.

Orphans should be kept in controlled heat of 80–90 degrees for the first 5 days. After this, drop the temperature gradually to about 80°. Use baby oil for dryness on the puppy's skin.

After feeding gently massage the puppy on the stomach and under the tail with wet cotton. This "burping" will aid in urination and defecation.

Colostrum, the milk produced over the first 24 hours, contains antibodies against distemper, hepatitis and other diseases. This immunity is passed on to the puppy. Depending upon the level of immunity existing in the mother these antibodies will gradually decrease over the next several months. For instance, it is possible to confer immunity against distemper to the puppies for 4 months through the colostrum, though 80–85% are free of the dam's protection by 9 weeks. Those not receiving this first 24 hours' milk have only limited immunity from the uterus, and can be vaccinated for distemper as early as 3 weeks of age. A continuous protection against distemper and hepatitis should be kept up until adult vaccinations are given (see section on vaccinations).

Puppy Disease

Puppies may get ill and succumb rapidly to disease. They have little resistance as they are using all their food and reserve to grow and meet their environmental challenge. The immunity received from the dam is a very important factor in their early survival.

The normal cardinal signs examined for illness are different in puppies than adults as the following indicates.

NORMAL PUPPIES

Heart Rate—200 min.—depending on breed

Respiration Rate—20–30 per minute

Temperature—100°

Mucous Membranes—pink but generally lighter than adults.

Skin—elastic, unwrinkled and springy.

SICK PUPPIES

Puppies which are wrinkled, cold and cry a lot are troubled. Those that are cold, clammy and quiet are in danger of dying.

Litters of puppies often fade away and die. This is called the "fading puppy syndrome." One puppy after another is found dead. The owner often thinks that the bitch has sat on them, but the dam is usually very careful and seldom kills one of her get. If a pup does not seem to be doing well or the dam rejects it, examine it carefully. If in doubt or if it seems very weak consult your veterinarian. If your litter is valuable each lost puppy is a blow to your pocket book. If a puppy fades and dies take the body to the veterinarian for immediate autopsy. Keep the puppy refrigerated until your veterinarian is available. It may be that examination of the rest of the litter is necessary or that laboratory work is necessary to pinpoint the cause. Using the right drug at this time is essential for the safety of the rest of the litter. Wide range antibiotics are usually employed either specifically or until laboratory results are at hand. Following are discussions on the different syndromes present in fading puppies.

Chilling is a prime cause of death. Pneumonia develops rapidly after chilling. Puppies that crawl away from the mother in a chilled environment may not live to see adulthood.

Virus is always a possibility. Great numbers of puppies succumb to distemper and hepatitis before reaching 6 months of age. At pre-weaning age they may die without any of the normal symptoms of these diseases. The viruses may be introduced from the environment, from visitors, or from the dam. Herpes virus causes generalized infection which usually ends in death in 24 hours. It is a relatively newly recognized disease of infant pups. Only an autopsy can differentiate this killer from any others. Bitches showing signs of vaginitis may be carriers of this disease. Treatment will help to prevent its occurence. After whelping once, the bitch may have a normal litter next time.

Pluero-pneumonia-like-organisms (PPLO's) also cause a sudden-death "fading syndrome" similar to the others.

Bacteria infection is acquired inter-uterine and causes abortion or early death of puppies. It may cause a clinical metritis in the bitch or may lie dormant until the next breeding. Other infections are acquired via the umbilical cord or orally after birth. These infections result in a variety of clinical pictures and include septicemia (generalized infection), navel illness or joint illness. Septicemia is a generalized infection in which lungs, liver, kidneys, heart or intestine or any other organ (or combination of organs) may be found infected at post mortem. *Escherichia coli* and *pseudomonas* bacteria commonly show a hemorrhagic enteritis on postmortem examination. Navel illness generally manifests itself as a hot, suppurative infection of the umbilicus and surrounding area. Streptococci and Staphylococci generally cause this type. Joint illness is usually a later infection. If the puppy survives the earlier attacks, the infection may lodge in the joints causing swelling and purulent closed joint infection. This infection site must be lanced and drained and treated with antibiotics.

Because all of these syndromes are similar and it may take several days to complete laboratory work, usually a generalized regime of treatment is undertaken until the laboratory report is in.

Your veterinarian will put the puppies on a wide-range antibiotic, one which he thinks will be of the most value. Usually he will inject the puppies with serum or globulum to give tham a passive immunity against distemper and hepatitis.

You should raise the temperature in the puppies' area to about 80 degrees if they are still with the mother, 90 degrees if not. Supplement feeding of the puppies, especially the weak ones. It is likely that you will need the stomach tube method for those unwilling to suckle. A few drops of raw liver juice added to the diet of each puppy at each feeding is advantageous. Puppies that survive the first 2 days have a good prognosis.

Congenital Malformations

Every puppy should be checked for malformations. Some of these will not show up for many weeks, others are immediately noticeable.

Cleft palates can be seen at birth.

Sometimes this even extends to include lip malformations. These puppies are difficult to raise and require surgery; they should be eliminated.

Hernias are sometimes obvious but usually not until the puppies are 3 or 4 weeks old. Umbilical hernias are most common and are easy to repair surgically. If small enough these hernias may close on their own when the whelps are about 6 months of age and be of no harm to the puppy. Puppies possessing umbilical hernia will tend to pass this fault to their get as it is highly hereditary. Ingrinal hernias are harder to find. Often small ones on bitches weak in the area do not show until pregnancy occurs. Then the hernia, which lies in the abdominal wall next to the thigh, will open and often enclose the gravid uterus and intestinal tract. Scrotal hernia in male puppies will often show very early. The scrotum looks as though the testicles are extra large, but careful checking will disclose that this bulk is frequently the intestinal tract. Both these hernias are surgically repairable but geneticists believe that they also are of hereditary origin.

Cryptorchids are dogs with one or both testicles contained in the body rather than in the scrotum. Monorchidism is not a proper medical term but a breeder's term to denote a single testicle retained.

The testicle begins its life in the same region as the ovary but during embryonic development it descends to the scrotum. A hereditary factor may cause retention of the testicle. If it remains in the abdominal cavity it becomes infertile due to temperature and developmental regression. These testicles have a greater tendency to become cancerous later in life than a normal testicle. If the testicle descends to the inguinal canal (the canal from the abdomen to the scrotum, parallel to the thigh), the dog may often be fertile while technically a cryptorchid. Check your puppy for testicles. The majority will have their testicles by 6 weeks. If not, get a guarantee that they will descend or do not take the puppy. The latest descend by 3 or $3\frac{1}{2}$ months but in rare cases it may take over 6 months. If your dog does not have both testicles by $3\frac{1}{2}$ months it is possible he will never have them. This condition is highly hereditary so be careful of litter brothers and sisters who may carry the recessive gene while being physically normal.

Congenital Heart Conditions

The incidence of congenital heart conditions may be as high as 5% but most cases that succumb early (post-natal) remain undiagnosed. Patent *ductus arteriosis* is the most common defect. It is a shunt between the aorta and pulmonary artery. It produces a machinery murmur in the stethoscope and a palpable thrill. Such pups tire easily and exhibit a blueness of the mucous membranes due to oxygen lack (*cyanosis*).

Persistant right aortic arch is a left over arch which usually disappears during embryonic development. This arch, the commonest, or a double aortic arch, or a malpositioned subclavian artery, may cross and cause varying amounts of compression of the esophagus. As the compression increases with growth, the puppy begins to vomit when attempting to eat solid foods.

Stenosis may occur on either side of the heart. Pulmonic stenosis is seen in the diagram and may be at the valve or in the body of the right ventricle. Aortic stenosis is only in the valvular area as the cavity of the left ventricle is larger and the walls are thinner, making it non-susceptible. Clinically the animals live longer than with the other defects and eventually show signs of general cardiac disease. Aortic stenosis is found most often in Boxers and German Shepherds.

Interventricular septal defect is an opening between the ventricles

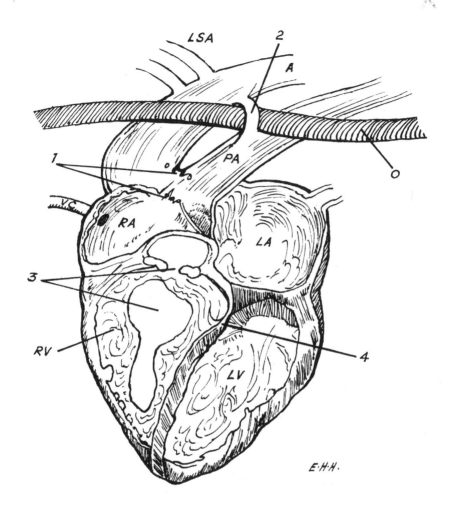

CUTAWAY OF CANINE HEART

A composite drawing of various congenital malformations which can occur in the puppy. 1. Patent ductus arteriosus 2. Persistent right aortic arch 3. Stenosis 4. Interventricular septal defect

A. Aorta PA. Pulmonary artery O. Oesphagus VC. Vena cava RA. Right auricle LA. Left auricle RV. Right ventricle LV. Left ventricle LSA. Left subclavicle artery

allowing the blood to flow back and forth. The condition produces a murmur and the dog shows signs of congestive heart failure.

Tetralogy of Fallot is a syndrome combining interventricle septal defect and pulmonic stenosis. These pups can tolerate very little exercise before turning cyanotic even as tiny puppies.

Only your veterinarian can find these congenital faults and some of them may not become evident because they are small or because they develop with growth such as the arch defects. If you can feel a definite trill under your fingers overriding the normal two beat heart pulse you may assume a heart condition is present.

Congenital Eye Problems

Entropian is an inversion of the eyelids. It may not show until the puppy is several months old. It causes mechanical conjunctivitis and results in infections and ulcers. It is particularly prevalent in certain breeds e.g.: Great Danes, Labrador Retrievers, and Norwegian Elkhounds.

Ectropian, the eversion of the lids, also causes *conjunctivitis* but is often a natural characteristic of certain breeds like Bassets and Bloodhounds. Both these conditions can be corrected surgically.

Congenital absence or malposition of the lacrimal openings (the lacrimal apparatus helps to produce and carry away tears) causes tearing and staining. Surgery can be employed to relieve the condition.

Congenital cataracts occur but they are rare. Often their removal by surgery can result in the return of good eyesight.

The retina (the area at the rear of the eye) suffers from many conditions. "*Collie eye*," which seldom causes complete blindness, is a retinal and optic disc degeneration which occurs in 50% of all Collies. Retinal detachment is seen most frequently in Bedlington Terriers and retinal atrophy in Irish Setters.

Bone Malformation

Congenital malformations of the vertebrae occur which result in kinked and compressed spinal columns. If not too extensive the dog may live a normal life. But the condition may cause motor and sensory nerve malfunctions. Intestinal or bladder control may be affected. Malformations of this type are most common in Bulldogs, Boston Terriers and terriers in general.

Congenital and hereditary malformations of the hip joint are common but not usually diagnosed until 6 months or over and even up to middle age.

They will be discussed in detail in the sections on muscular-skeletal diseases.

Stockard's Syndrome

Stockard's Syndrome is an inherited condition caused by a triple set of dominant genes. It usually occurs at 3 months of age but it can manifest itself at from 2 to 4 months. Basically it is a motor neuron degeneration in the lumbar section of the spinal cord. It is most common in Great Danes, Bloodhounds, St. Bernards and in interbred specimens of these breeds.

The condition manifests itself as a partial or complete paralysis and atrophy of the hind legs with the legs in extension. There is no known treatment nor does the animal get better.

Imperfect apposition of the teeth

Overshot jaw (parrot mouth) occurs when the upper jaw overhangs the lower jaw. Undershot jaw (Bulldog mouth) is when the lower jaw protrudes beyond the upper jaw.

Undershot jaws are natural in some breeds, e.g. Boxers, Bulldogs, Shih Tzus and Bostons. When these conditions exist except in breeds where it is natural, the dog is considered unsound. The conditions are inherited as a recessive.

The sicssors bite
(correct for most breeds)

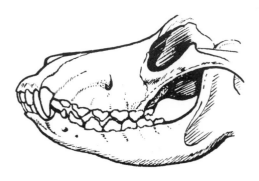
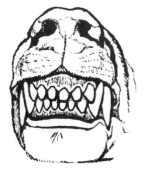

Hydrocephalus

A hydrocephalic puppy has excessive amounts of cerebrospinal fluid. The animal will have an enlarged head. These animals may also have open fontanelles. The condition is usually congenital but may be acquired as a secondary effect of tumor or meningitis.

The dog shows depression, incoordination and possibly has convulsions.

Soft Spots

A soft spot in the skull is called a fontanel. It is an unossified area between the bone sutures in the skull. Animals with this anomaly can show similar symptoms to a hydrocephalic puppy and are subject to injury.

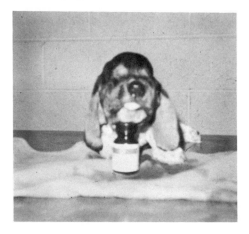

A HYDROCEPHALIC PUPPY
Half of the skull of this Bassett puppy was missing, causing a swollen, fluid-filled area under the skin.

Tail Docking

Docking is usually done at 2 to 3 days of age although it can be done as early as 24 hours after birth. Following is a list of standard lengths. It will be seen that this may vary in some breeds with breeder or show trends. For instance, Springer Spaniel owners of field stock usually want as little as $\frac{1}{3}$ of the tail removed. Germans often dock Schnauzer tails shorter than the American trend. This is something that has often been done by breeders but if you have not had experience docking do not try it as I have seen puppies bleed to death when docking is attempted by the inexperienced amateur.

Tail Lengths

Welsh, Irish, Lakeland, Kerry Blue, Wire Fox, West Highland White, Smooth Fox, Sealyham, Airedale—Terriers—leave $\frac{1}{2}$ tail.

Norwich Terrier, Yorkshire Terrier, Brittany Spaniel, Brussels Griffon—leave $\frac{1}{3}$ tail.

Cocker Spaniel, English Cocker Spaniel, English Toy Spaniel,

Welsh Corgi—leave $\frac{1}{4}$ tail.

Affenpinscher, Schipperke, Rottweiler, Old English Sheepdog—leave $\frac{1}{4}$ inch.

Poodles—all sizes—leave $\frac{2}{3}$ tail.

Miniature Pinscher—leave $\frac{1}{2}$ inch.

Boxer—$\frac{3}{4}$ inch—but may vary with breeder or style.

Giant Schnauzer—1 inch but may vary with breeder or style.

Miniature Schnauzer—1 inch but may vary with breeder or style.

Standard Schnauzer—1 inch but may vary with breeder or style.

Doberman Pinscher—$\frac{1}{2}$ inch but may vary with breeder or style.

German Shorthaired Pointer—leave $\frac{1}{3}$ but may vary with breeder or style.

Weimaraner—leave $\frac{1}{4}$ length but may vary with breeder or style.

The length of tail left after docking varies greatly according to breed. It is a job that requires expertise, so leave it to your veterinarian. The docked pup is a Schnauzer.

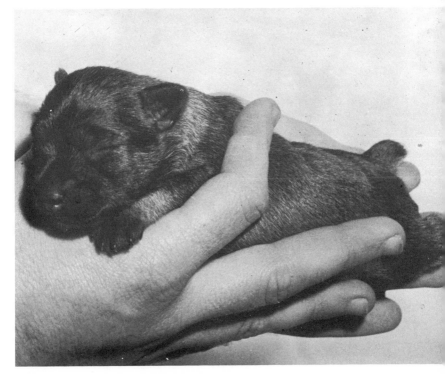

Cropping

Ear cropping is usually done at 8 — 12 weeks but larger breeds may be done earlier and smaller breeds can wait for several months. The Boston Terrier is one breed that can have natural bat ears or be cropped. In England cropping is not allowed and domestic dogs which are cropped are unshowable. This law exists in many of our states. It is archaic as it has never stopped cropping. Instead it has created a group of non-professional men known as "croppers." These people do so many ears a year that they become excellent technicians at fashioning the correct breed pattern but most have little or no knowledge of aseptics and can do a crude and painful job. As the laws change these individuals are becoming a vanishing breed like the dinosaur. Therefore, if you want a particular pattern bring pictures and drawings and discuss the crop with your veterinarian; he will be happy to work with you.

A seven weeks old Great Dane puppy before cropping. Note the spread of the youngster's ears, indicative of its "Boarhound" origin.

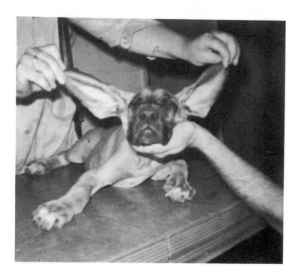

Dewclaws

Dewclaws are removed on many breeds for two purposes. Hunting breeds and those breeds requiring constant clipping and grooming have them removed to avoid injury. The most common reason for

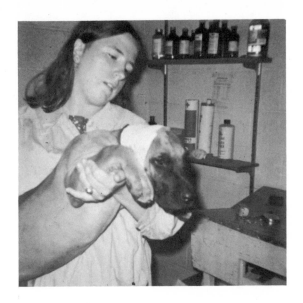

The same seven weeks old Great Dane puppy
immediately after cropping, wearing
a "bonnet."

A few days following surgery, the puppy has
his ears taped into natural position to
help train the muscles to hold them correctly.

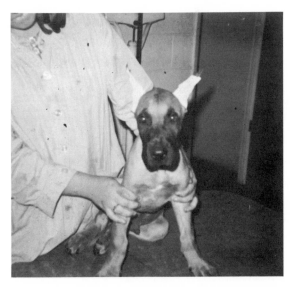

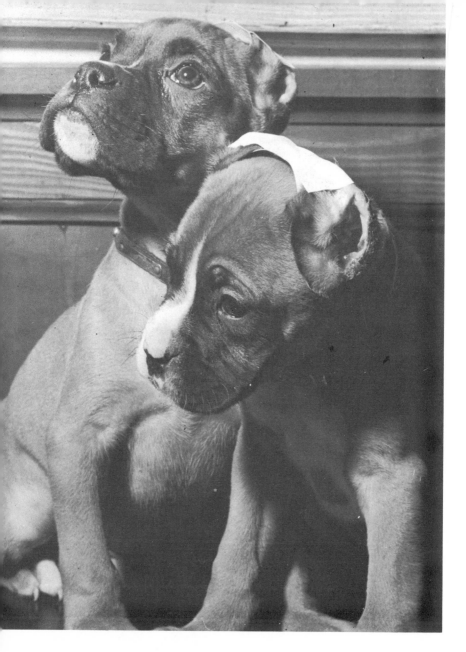

Your Boxer puppy's ears should be cropped when
the pup is seven or eight weeks of age. Have a
veterinarian do the job. The ears should be taped
afterward and the tape left on as long as advised.

78

removal is to present a clean leg for dog shows. Care must be taken to consult your standard before removal because there are exceptions. While it is a fault to heave rear dewclaws in most breeds, in Great Pyrenees and Briards it is required that they have double rear dewclaws and in St. Bernards it is optional.

German Shepherds should never have front dewclaws removed but should have rear ones taken off if present.

They are removed when puppies are between 24 hours to 4 days old as the best time. It is not improper to allow front dewclaws to remain in any breed but you may be a "frowned upon amateur" in the show ring when your dog is shown.

Coprophagy

Stool eating is common in puppies. It is a result of boredom. The habit usually disappears with maturity. Cleaning the runs and removal of all stools is a practice of prime importance.

Staph (acne)—This is a common puppy skin infection in the facial area. (See pyoderma—skin disease section.)

Toxic Thymus

The *Thymus* is a gland lying in the proximal chest area. As yet the purpose or job of this gland is unknown. It degenerates as the dog grows. There is a condition of unknown etiology in puppies 3 weeks to 3 months old where the thymus becomes enlarged, causing diffisulty in breathing and sudden deaths. Corticosteroids are the treatment of choice at the moment.

Scottie Cramp

Scottie cramp is an inherited muscular condition of Scottish Terriers of about 2 weeks or older.

It appears in healthy dogs during exercise. The muscles of the hind end become rigid and the dog "bunny" hops. This spreads to the forelimbs if exercise is continued. The condition usually will not recur if exercise is curtailed and not forced.

Hysteria

Hysteria occurs when external pressures cause the dog to exceed the brain threshold over which he cannot exist in a normal state. This can be considered "an overload of the circuits." The result is a motor fit or a hysterical dog.

The puppy may be born with a low threshold and thus be an epileptic, or it may have a threshold lowered from disease. Distemper and encephalitis can cause permanent brain damage resulting in just such a problem. The dog can exceed a normal threshold due to parasites, calcium deficiency, some foods, internal discomfort, foreign bodies or ear mites.

The convulsion will last a few seconds to a $\frac{1}{2}$ hour. It can be accompanied by partial paralysis, or running, or coma.

Patterns are often established so the owner should keep track of all environmental stimuli prior to the occurrence.

These dogs are treated with epileptiform drugs.

Hypoglycemia in puppies

This condition occurs mainly in toy breeds between 6 and 12

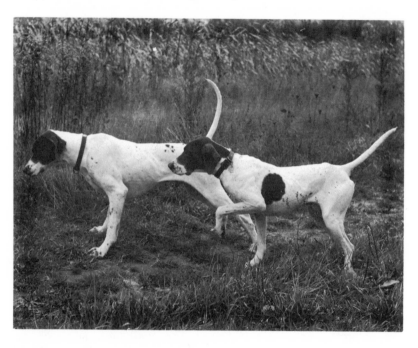

A condition similar to hypoglycemia (seen usually
in toy breed puppies) also occurs in adult
hunting dogs, usually when working in the field.

weeks of age. It is precipitated by stress. The puppy has excess glycogen stored in the body depots but is unable to utilize it to produce glucose; thus one of the body's major metabolic cycles is broken down. The blood sugar is low (hypoglycemia). Under stress the puppies exhibit incoordination, sunken eyes, depression and muscle tremors. This continues into coma and finally death.

Therapy is directed at restoring blood levels of glucose and stimulating glycogen usage through corticosteroid therapy.

Owners of toy puppies should not overtire them and should see that they eat at least every 8 hours. In kennels where this occurs with any frequency the breeding program should be carefully examined.

A similar condition occurs in adult hunting dogs usually when hunting. Care should be taken to feed these dogs before hunting and to increase the animal protein in their diet.

With proper diet both groups, puppies and adult hunting dogs,

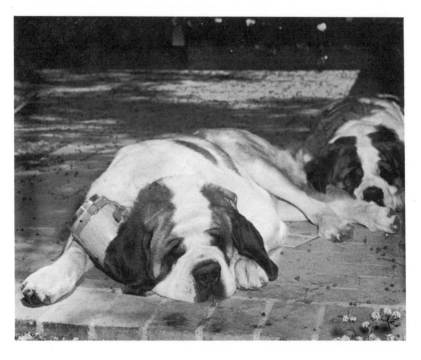

Because of their tremendous growth, dogs of giant breeds, such as the St. Bernards pictured above, are prone to dietary deficiency diseases.

have a good prognosis for control.

Rickets

Rickets occurs in growing puppies. It is a deficiency disease caused by a group of conditions.

1. Low vitamin D. Vitamin D is needed by the animal's body to

utilize calcium. Even with excess calcium if vitamin D is deficient the dog will show evidence of rickets. Most of the needed vitamin D is supplied by sunlight, therefore puppies raised indoors have a greater tendency toward rickets. Oils tend to reduce vitamin D utilization.

Calcium is needed in certain minimal amounts by the body in order to form proper bone growth. It is supplied through good diet and supplementation.

Phosphorus must be in a certain ratio of calcium to phosphorus (1.2 to 1). Too much phosphorus will cause hypocalcium in the dog even though the calcium supplementation is high.

The dog shows bowing of the limbs and knobby joints. This is caused by lack of calcification in the metaphysis (the growing area between the shaft and the heads of the long bones). The bones are soft and may fracture. The dog is often lame, "down in the pasterns" and shows a row of knobs along the ends of the ribs.

Diagnosis is usually easily made upon clinical appearance but can be confirmed by X-ray and calcium/phosphorus blood levels.

Treatment and prevention is in proper diet and supplementation of vitamin D, calcium and phosphorus. Small breeds are less sus-

Normal front

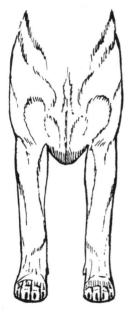

Rickets

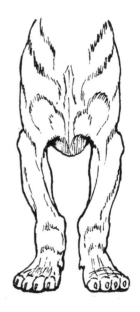

ceptible to clinical rickets as the ratio of weight to leg strength and bone capable of supporting the body is not as far apart as it is in giant breeds like Great Danes. Doses as high as 300 units vitamin D per lb. may be advisable in large breeds particularly during the winter months. Calcium rich foods, such as milk, are excellent as are bone meal and prepared calcium supplements. The calcium content of giant and heavy breeds should be approximately 1% of the wet weight of the food while .5% is normal for lighter breeds. Thus, since most commercial foods when wet contain about .4% calcium minimal supplements, the requirement for most breeds, in heavy and giant breeds up to 60% calcium may have to be added. Working on the basis of 240 mg. of calcium per pound of body weight of a growing giant breed it can be computed that a 30 lb. Great Dane puppy needs 7.2 grams of calcium. A good commercial food will supply 3.6 grams on the average so that 3.6 grams (or approximately 55 grains) must be added at the upper limits. Considering the weight of your dog, the breed, and the content of your supplement, it should be easy to feed the proper amount of calcium.

Diets rich in phosphorus should contain supplements that are not completely calcium diphosphate. Grains and cereals are commonly higher in phosphorus than calcium so this should be taken into consideration.

It should also be remembered that as the dog gets close to total growth, the calcium supplementation should reduce closer to maintenance (.5% of diet). Therefore, a balance between weight and age should be reached and the calcium should not be continually increased. As an example the author has seen Dane puppies raised with great success on a maximum of 75 grains of calcium additive in a good diet.

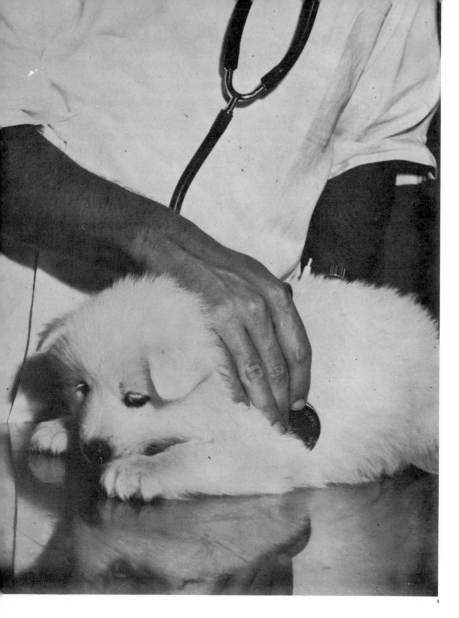

Over the years deadly infectious diseases have taken their toll of canine lives. Intense research has uncovered causes and aided in recognition of these vicious microscopic killers. Control, treatment, and immunization are offered by your veterinarian in the constant fight against these lethal diseases.

84

CHAPTER 6

INFECTIOUS DISEASES

Viral Disease

In the category of infectious diseases we find the dreaded viral and bacterial, spirochetal and fungus diseases, caused by the activity of vicious microscopic organisms that over the years have taken their dread toll of canine life.

Luckily intense and successful research by dedicated veterinarians and scientists over a long period of time has resulted in an understanding and definite recognition of these diseases and the eventual discovery of various elements, agents, and specific medications useful in controlling, treating, and immunizing our dogs against the lethal attacks of these tiny, insidious, cripplers and killers.

Distemper (*Carre's disease*)

This is the dread disease of dogs. Of all the diseases and catastrophies known, distemper kills or maims more dogs than any other. Although the puppy, exposed and unprotected, is as a group the hardest hit, this disease is not limited to the young. It can attack with just as much virulence a dog of any age. Immunity, whether by vaccination or environment, is not life-long (see chapter on immunity and vaccination).

So often I hear "This dog nevèr had shots, Doc, and he is healthier than any of those fancy pure-bred dogs." This is a misconception. The animal usually is the sole survivor of a large family whose medical history is lost with their early, unattended deaths. These are the forgotten dogs that died of "worms," whose mother "lay" on them, or they "disappeared," were "stolen" or "poisoned," but that probably really succumbed to distemper early in life. The present live pet usually survives with an immunity which is periodically revitalized through constant contact in his unhealthy environment. Today we are interested in life, not death, so our aims are to raise and protect every life we can and not leave it to nature to pick a lucky 5 or 10% for survival in every litter.

The virus of distemper attacks particular cells which line the lungs, intestine and brain, and are present in other organs. Thus we have widespread symptoms and effects upon the dog. The incubation period is 7 to 20 days after contact.

In a typical clinical case, the dog starts with a temperature rise, goes off his feed and becomes lethargic. The temperature drops to normal for a few days, but the dog begins to show upper respiratory problems, such as moist eyes and nose. Diarrhea and vomiting develop next, either with or followed by pneumonia and coughing. The temperature is back up. Secondary invasion of bacteria occurs turning the eye and nose discharges to pus. The dog is spreading the disease through its infected body discharges, and the virus, which is very resistant, has been known to survive in the environment for up to 6 months. The virus can also travel by wind currents, contaminated clothing and shoes, and contaminated dog equipment. Skin infection of the stomach and thighs is another secondary common infection. Gradually, after the first week or two, nervous changes may develop. The symptoms may delay for several weeks even after the dog has shown clinical recovery. The dog may show nervous defects ranging from blindness, paralysis, muscle tremors (chorea), and hysteria, to convulsions in the encephalitic (brain) form. If the dog survives long enough "hard pad" changes develop which cause the feet to become like linoleum in texture.

The puppy may succumb to dehydration, lack of nutrition and shock early in the disease, but most older dogs die of the encephalitic effects or an uncontrolled secondary infection. Mortality is very high.

Treatment consists of supplying as much nourishment and fluids as possible, antibiotics for secondary disease control, antidistemper serums to attack the virus early in the disease, vitamins and good nursing.

Prevention from distemper is the most important thing we can do for a dog. Your dog is never too young nor too old to be protected. A planned protective program should be started or planned from birth and carried out through life. Measurement of the mother's immunity will help the veterinarian to plan puppy vaccination, or use of serums that will protect the youngster until it is old enough

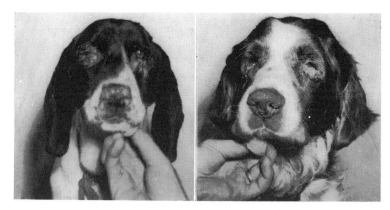

These two dogs are exhibiting all the signs of infection by the dread viral distemper (Carre's disease). This virus is widespread.

to vaccinate. Most puppies can use a vaccine by 9 weeks of age, having been brought to this age through the use of serums or other control methods. All puppies can be vaccinated by four months of age, but if we wait until then many would fall victim to the disease. Set up your program with your veterinarian immediately upon acquiring your puppy or upon the birth of a litter. (See Immunity and Vaccination.)

Some authorities have attempted to segregate other diseases from distemper and give them individual importance such as, the "show dog" disease of the early part of the century, "house dog" disease, hard-pad disease or encephalitis. Most of these have never been scientifically proven to be separate diseases and are just manifestations of true distemper in a milder or non-symptomatic form. The clinical picture described earlier occurs only part of the time. Many dogs show only mild signs or only some of the symptoms, thus causing confusion in diagnosis and an attempt to create new diseases to fit the symptoms. Encephalitis exists as a primary entity beyond doubt, but it is most common as a part of distemper. Stamp out this canine killer. Vaccinate!

Infectious Canine Hepatitis (*Rubarth's disease*)

This condition was first separated from distemper by full scientific investigation in the late forties, thus eliminating many of the earlier problems in vaccine and disease understanding.

The virus attacks the cells of the liver and causes temperature and

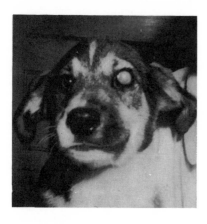

Clinical picture of a dog after contracting infectious canine hepatitis. This virus attacks the cells of the liver.

mucous membrane congestion. The disease may be acute or sub-acute, or even sub-clinical. The incubation period is about one week after contact. Acute cases show high temperature rise, abdominal pain and sudden death.

Sub-clinical cases may show a temperature rise if the temperature is taken at the right time but, since death is almost nil, the only way of knowing that the dog was infected is from the presence of immunity bodies known to have been produced by the disease, or the appearance of a "blue eye" (corneal opacity) seven to ten days after the disease subsides. This latter lesion is considered confirmation of the diagnosis.

In the sub-acute, or more common disease form, the dog shows a high temperature rise, abdominal pain in the liver area, vomiting, and often enlarged tonsils. The dog may develop hemorrhages in the skin or mucous membranes, swelling from fluids in the head, neck and body, and jaundice. The mortality rate is between 10 to 30%.

During the disease phase the virus is found throughout the body but after recovery it remains in the kidneys for many months making the urine a source of infection to other dogs. Fortunately the virus cannot survive for too many hours in the normal environment.

Upon post-mortem, hepatitis dogs show swollen, congested livers, and enlarged and congested gall bladders.

Treatment early in the disease is accomplished through serums to fight the virus. Usually mixed distemper-hepatitis serums are used because diagnosis could be confused early and useless later, after the disease has progressed to the point of positive identification. Antibiotics are given to avoid secondary infections. Vitamin B complex and drugs that bring digestive relief and help the liver to relax are part of the treatment. Good, high quality protein and low fat diets are helpful, as well as careful, general nursing.

Once again vaccination is the prevention, "an ounce of prevention is worth a pound of cure" and is less expensive than treating the disease.

Rabies

Rabies is a viral disease affecting the brain in all mammals, including man. Once the symptoms have started death is the normal outcome. The state-sponsored rabies programs and information services have done much to control the disease and eradicate it from our pets. Vaccination is essential in areas where the disease is endemic, and always wise anywhere in the USA.

The virus, which is present in the animal's saliva, enters via a bite (or other) wound. The virus then travels via a series of nerves to the brain, after which the typical symptoms develop.

Incubation is usually 15 days to a month, but there have been rare cases recorded in which the virus took several months to incubate. The virus travels from the brain again via a nerve to enter the saliva. This occurs only a few days before clinical onset of the disease, therefore, observation of a dog for 10–15 days after it has inflicted a bite is necessary to be sure it could not have transferred the disease. If any dog dies after biting within the 10 day period it is wise, especially in any area where rabies has been reported, to have the brain examined. Your veterinarian or Public Health official will advise you on the proper procedure.

It has also been found in some instances, specifically in small enclosed areas where contamination is heavy, that the infection can be airborne. This has been shown experimentally but, except perhaps for caves containing infected bats, this method of infectivity probably plays no part in the normal pattern. Bats have been found rabid in better than half the states and are a reservoir of infection constantly ready to challenge the outside world.

The first sign is a change in behavior. Excess saliva may or may not be produced at this time. Usually the rabid victims stop eating and drinking and seek quiet, dark places. There is often increased urination and sexual desire. After a few days the animals resent handling and go either into the paralytic or furious form.

In the paralytic form the animal's muscles around the head become paralyzed and the jaw hangs. Excess salivation occurs. Paralysis continues to increase, leading to coma and death.

The furious form is the "mad dog" form so often written of in literature. Here the dog is aggressive, the face is tense and shows anxiety, the pupils dilate and the dog attacks moving objects. The infected animal is excited and is not aware of fear or enemies. These are the vicious and deadly roamers which attack other animals, people, or anything that moves. As the condition progresses, incoordination and convulsions occur and finally death.

There is no cure once symptoms have begun. Vaccination is the prevention. The vaccines utilized are both of the live and killed varieties. Killed vaccines confer an immunity for one year while live vaccines may immunize for up to 3 years.

Bacterial Diseases

Any pathogenic bacteria can cause non-specific bacterial infection known as a *septicemia* or *bacteremia*, In bacteremia the blood contains circulating bacteria or its toxins. The infection enters at a certain focal point, often from a localized infection which becomes generalized. Thus an abcess may lose its solitary local infection form and infect the entire body causing temperature rise and a multitude of symptoms, depending upon the areas most affected. Listlessness, chills, infected membranes and a rise in white blood cells are also general changes. Positive identification of such an infection lies in taking and examining cultures either from the source area or blood.

Antibiotics are the basic attacking force. Where the exact nature of the bacteria is unknown, wide-range antibiotics or combinations are often employed.

Tetanus

Tetanus is a specific bacterial disease caused by *Clostridium tetani*. The bacteria enter a wound and grow but do not invade the body system. The total body effects are caused by toxins produced by the bacteria. Tetanus bacteria grow best where there is a lack of oxygen, therefore puncture wounds are the most dangerous.

Tetanus is not a common disease in dogs that have, as a species, a natural resistance to the bacteria, but nevertheless it should never be discarded.

The dog shows stiffness and nervousness. Gradually the animal indicates increased hypersensitivity to noise and touch. Spasms of convulsion-like stiffness occur. Temperature rises. Finally the respiratory muscles are effected and death ensues.

Tetanus may be confused with strichnine poisoning but with tetanus the onset is more gradual and the spasms more lasting. The animal's clinical history may also help differentiate.

Treatment is with high doses of tetanus antitoxin. Penicillin helps to kill the bacteria. Locating and cleaning the original wound site is also helpful. Sedatives relieve the symptomatic pain.

Prevention can be by vaccine but this is not commonly practiced in dogs. Cleaning wounds and administering tetanus antitoxin when necessary will almost invariably prevent the infection.

Brucellosis

It has become apparent that the Brucella species bacteria can infect dogs. These bacteria cause genital disease in cows, pigs and sheep as well as general disease. The dog contacts the infection by eating contaminated material, e.g. the farm dog devours the placenta of a Brucellae aborted calf, etc.

The organism causes granulomas and abcesses in lymph nodes, liver, kidney and spleen. Infections of the testes is common and abortion in bitches has been noted. The dog shows an undulating temperature and often painful movement.

The diagnosis can be made from a blood titer.

Use of wide-range antibiotics is the recommended treatment.

Tularemia

Tularemia is a Pasteurella bacterial infection mainly of rodents to which the dog is only mildly susceptible. Transmission can result by contact with open wounds and from biting insects. It causes many small areas of infection in the lungs, liver, spleen, lymph nodes and kidney. This leaves the dog susceptible to pneumonia and degeneration of the organs involved.

The symptoms often resemble distemper, with fever, vomiting, and loss of appetite. The blood picture shows a definite bacterial infection and the area where the disease enters often becomes ulcerated and itchy.

The disease runs a course of three weeks with slow but spontaneous recovery. Streptomycin, chloromycetin, and aueromycin are all helpful.

Listerellosis

Listerella monocytogenes affects all domestic animals. It affects the nervous system as well as causing pneumonia and bacteremia.

The infected dog shows abnormal temperature, circling, convulsions and finally death. Pneumonia is present in some victims. Mortality is almost 100% in spite of treatment attempts with numerous antibiotics.

Listeria have also been found as a low grade uterine infection causing "fading puppies," infertility and abortion.

Tuberculosis

Mycobacterium tuberculosis is an infectious disease of domestic animals and man. The pet dog, most usually contacts it from an infected person in the household, or from infected milk. The animal then becomes a source of infection, especially to the close child companion. Fortunately it is a rare disease of dogs in the United States.

The condition has a slow, insidious onset with a chronic course. Because of this, the dog is seldom seen by the veterinarian until it is in the advanced stages. The dog has gradually lost weight, exhibits hard breathing and a chronic cough. X-rays of the lungs often show TB lesions. Some cases are alimentary in nature with depleting diarrhea. If this infection is suspected all efforts at identification should be made.

Because of the possibility of infection spread and the difficulty in successful treatment in dogs, euthanasia is advisable.

Spirochetal Diseases

Only two diseases of the spirochetal bacteria are of any importance. The first is Trench Mouth, and the second, Leptospirosis.

Canine Trench Mouth

Trench Mouth is a gum infection of dogs caused by a spirochete and a fusiform organism; it is not uncommon. Vitamin B and C deficiencies and diseased teeth predispose the dog to infection.

The dog has bad breath with ulceration and degeneration of the gums. The organism can be identified in smears.

Treatment consists of treating predisposing causes, using antibiotics, especially penicillin, and antiseptic mouth paints.

Leptospirosis (*Weil's or Stuttgart's disease*)

The two varieties of Leptospirosis which affect dogs are *Leptospira canicola* and *Leptospira icterohemorrhagiae.* While *L. icterohemorrhagiae* is common to many animals, basically only man and dog are infected by *L. canicola.* The spirochete is easily killed by heat or disinfectants but will survive in water or sewage for a long time. The main mode of transfer is via the urine. *Canicola* is usually transferred dog to dog or dog to man from contaminated food or handling of the urine. Besides oral infection it can enter through cuts and abrasions.

Icterohemorrhagiae usually is brought into the environment via a rat carrier. These animals only suffer mildly from the disease and can, after recovery, remain carriers for several years.

Clinically the dog shows varied symptoms which are affected by the fact that the condition can have an acute to chronic pattern. In general the dog shows inappetence and depression. The coat is dry. The animal often moves tucked up with choppy steps because of pain in the kidney area. The temperature is elevated, often to 106°. The gums and other mucous membranes are congested and may even become jaundiced. Vomiting is common, which may be bile or brown stained. As dehydration sets in, the urine becomes concentrated and dark yellow. Protein content of the urine is high. At times diarrhea occurs which may become bloody. If toxicity sets in nervous twitchings, or even convulsions, can occur.

The spirochete attacks especially the kidney and liver. Disease is also present in the intestinal tract and pleura and peritoneum.

Clinically the *canicola* disease is more concentrated in the kidneys and milder, while the *icterohemorrhagiae* produces more hemorrhage, greater liver as well as kidney damage, and is more severe than *canicola.*

Clinical examination followed by laboratory tests will confirm the diagnosis. This condition can be confused with hepatitis in its early stages. In leptospirosis the white blood cell count rises and the red blood cells fall, while the plasma is jaundiced. The BUN (blood-urea-nitrogen) will rise, especially in chronic cases. The spirochete can often be found in urine samples under the microscope using dark field examination. Serological tests will also help to confirm the diagnosis.

Treatment is with antibiotics, especially Streptomycin and some of the wide-range antibiotics. Immunity serum is also excellent. Couple the treatment with good, general nursing, similar care to that given the dog with kidney disease.

Recovery is always slow. Many cases become uremic or are predisposed to nephritis in later life because of kidney scarring. Recovered dogs can become carriers for long periods.

The disease can be prevented by vaccination. This is usually combined with your distemper-hepatitis program by your veterinarian and is a killed bi-valent vaccine.

Rickettsial Disease

These are a group of organisms existing between the bacteria and the viruses which use insects and snakes and flukes as transport hosts.

Salmon poison—This is not a poisoning but an infectious disease caused by a rickettsia which uses salmon and its parasites as the transport host. It is most common at salmon spawning time. The fish contains a small fluke parasite which harbors the rickettsia. The dog eats the fish containing the fluke containing the germ, thus ingesting the rickettsia.

The condition is common where salmon are found, especially from Northwest California and points north.

The disease starts suddenly with a temperature rise, the appetite is off and the animal listless. The high temperature is typical, reaching a peak of 104° to 106° in about 2 days and remaining high for several days. On the 6th to 8th day the temperature drops to normal or below. Death occurs a few days later. Diarrhea is common after a few days, becoming yellow and bloody in a short time. Vomiting also occurs and thirst is extreme.

Diagnosis is based on the symptoms, the area where the disease occurs, and the finding of fluke eggs in the feces.

Prevention is arrived at by simply not allowing the animal to eat raw salmon. While no vaccines have been developed survivors have a high level of immunity.

Treatment is with sulfonamides. Other wide-range antibiotics are also used with success.

Few other rickettsias have been identified in dogs, and most of them have no clinical importance.

Mycotic Diseases (*Fungus diseases*)

Fungus diseases are rarer than bacterial or viral disease and are usually identified with tropical areas. But with the great movement of animals throughout the world today they are becoming

94

more prevalent in other climes. They are difficult to treat and often overlooked in diagnosis.

Nocardiosis

This fungus is occasionally found in dogs. It most likely enters from the soil via the respiratory tract. Man is susceptible to infection but transmission has not been proved. The lung is infected and appears on X-ray much like TB, but the course of the disease is often acute with temperature and general weakness. Difficulty in breathing is marked. Chronic cases resemble TB with lung abcesses.

Wide range antibiotics and sulfonamides should be used in high doses, although definite scientific proof of a cure is not recorded.

Cryptococcosis

While this fungus can infect all organs, it has an affinity for the brain. Usually the condition is chronic, often lasting over a year. The dog loses weight, changes personality and may show nervous derangement. The result is usually death.

Moniliasis

Moniliasis is caused by *Candida albicans*. The fungus affects man and animals but is not contagious except perhaps by direct contact. It is a local or general infection of the skin and/or the mucous membranes and is usually not serious. Often a whitish film is present over the inflamed areas.

The application of wet packs of 1% crystal violet results in a good response from the patient.

Blastomycosis

Blastomyces dermatitides causes pustular granulomatous lesions especially on the skin, the lungs and bones. The condition has been reported in the southwestern United States. It causes two syndromes: the generalized systemic disease and the cutaneous form. The systemic form is slow spreading with a course of several months. It affects the lungs and/or the bones, accompanied by respiratory distress or swelling of the limbs. The cutaneous form shows crusty, purulent lesions which spread by contact.

There is no known effective treatment and the disease is a public health hazard to man.

Histoplasmosis

Histoplasma capsulatum is a progressive, rare disease with a high mortality rate which attacks humans and dogs.

The dog exhibits fever, anemia, low white blood cell count, en-

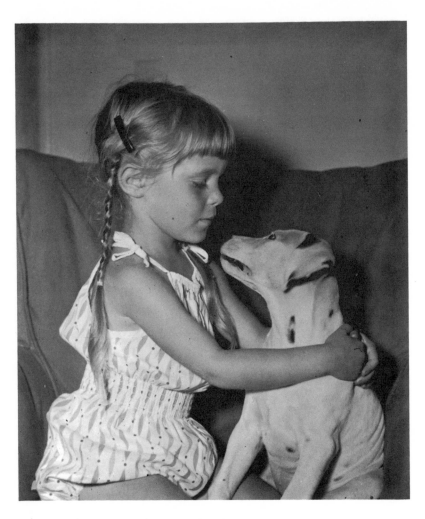

Most canine diseases cannot be communicated to man. But there are a few that can, and some canine diseases (histoplasmosis) have been associated with the same disease in children. Regular checkups by your veterinarian will alleviate any anxiety you may have.

larged spleen, loss of weight and, sometimes, diarrhea. The disease in dogs has been associated with the same disease in children.

Coccidioidomycosis

This fungus, while reported only occasionally, is probably the most common of the fungus diseases. It is caused by the fungus *Coccidioides immitis* (unrelated to protozoal coccidiosis).

It usually manifests itself as a self-limiting pulmonary infection found in dry dusty areas of the southwestern United States.

The symptoms vary with the severity of the cases. Mortality is low. The dog shows mild respiratory infection signs. The disease is suspected when a respiratory infection remains unchanged for several weeks and the area is hot and dry. X-rays, high eosinophils*, and an increased sedimentation rate in the blood count suggests the disease. A skin sensitivity test is available which aids in diagnosis but may show false negatives. Culturing will help to identify the organism.

While the disease is self-limiting in dogs, it is contagious to humans so that euthanasia is often recommended.

Aspergillosis

Aspergillus, fungus found in dry feed and grass, has caused rare respiratory infections.

Madura Foot

Madura foot is a granulomatous or ulcerative condition of the surface of the legs or feet of dogs. It is very rare. Hormodendrum (spp.) fungus causes the condition. Surgical removal or topical fungicides may control the condition but complete cure is difficult.

In general, it is to be noted that new fungicides are becoming available that may change the prognosis of many of these fungal diseases. Amphotericin B (*Fungizone*) is being used against Coccidioidomycosis, Histoplasmosis, Cryptococcosis and Blastomycosis. Griseofulvin is being recommended for Moniliasis and Madura Foot. Data about these drugs and their effects on dogs for these diseases is lacking at this time.

*A particular white blood cell, usually low in numbers.

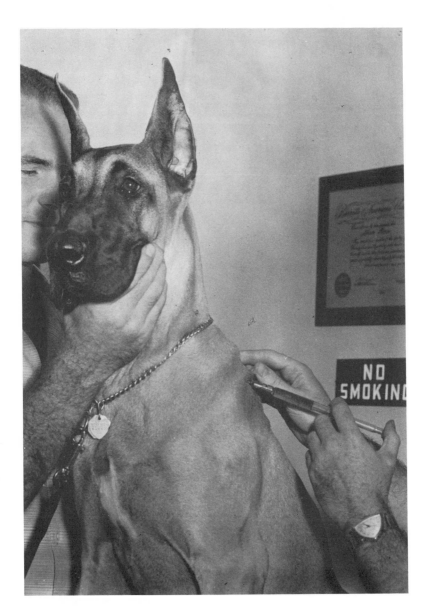

Resistance to disease is the most important
weapon the canine has to fight against illness.
Immunity through vaccination is a prime factor in
bringing this resistance to your dog. A vaccination
program should be set up by your veterinarian
to protect your dog's health.

CHAPTER 7

IMMUNITY AND VACCINATIONS

One of the most important weapons that the animal body possesses to protect itself against disease is "immunity." To understand immunity and how it is produced is perhaps the most important single piece of knowledge that the reader can gain from this book.

Literally *immunity* means complete protection, but medically the working definition is a *resistance to disease*. Protection is gained through "antibodies" which are anti-disease units produced by the body in response to an attack on the body by a particular disease unit, the antigen. These antibodies circulate in the body fluids, especially the blood stream, in association with serum globulin. The antibody is a specific unit which protects only against the specific antigen whose attack brought it into being. Microorganisms and their toxic products, or foreign proteins, are antigens which stimulate antibody production. Antibodies are produced through the reticulo-endothelial system, a system of disease destroying cells located in many organs of the body.

The known antibodies act in several ways:

1. *Antitoxins chemically neutralize toxins.*

2. *Precipitins (antibody) precipitate and thereby change proteins (antigen).*

3. *Agglutins causes a clumping of bacterial cells thus making physical spread difficult.*

4. *Lysins dissolve cells.*

5. *Opsonins stimulate destruction of antigens by the white blood cells.*

It is likely that there are other antibodies and antibody actions present in the blood which have not yet been discovered.

Immunity occurs also on the cellular level where cells become able to block the entrance of the antigen. This can be accomplished without known change to the body fluids.

While in most cases immunity can be measured by the amount of antibody present in the blood, in some cases immunity exists without measurable levels in the body fluids.

The amount of immunity which an animal will build up from antigen invasion depends upon the ability of the animal to build an immunity, blocking of the antigen by antibodies already present, and the ability of the antigen to stimulate immunity. So far as is known no immunity is life-time but wears out according to the foregoing factors. A dog receiving "lifetime" immunity must be figured against the length of the animal's lifetime. If he lived long enough the immunity would fade.

In *some* cases, after antibodies have been built up to a certain level, a second dose of antigen will cause an anamnestic reaction where the effect is a faster and higher rise in antibody level.

Therefore, when the animal's body is attacked by a virus or bacteria, he has two defense systems. First, the physical defenses of skin, tears, gastric juices, etc. which may all kill the invader, and second, his level of immunity against the invader.

The Production of Immunity

The dog may have either an inherent immunity or an acquired one. The inherent immunity may be on the species level (dogs do not get measles), or breed level (very little has been done on dogs in this field), or individual level.

Inherent immunity is of minor importance in most dog diseases. Acquired immunity is the more important type of immunity when weighing vaccination programs against the common diseases of dogs. It is divided into two categories, active and passive.

Passive immunity is only a temporary immunity. It consists of antibodies given to one dog from a second dog which has built up the antibody. Natural, passive immunity is passed to puppies from the uterus and the first 24 hour milk of the dam. This may have an effect of from 3 weeks to 4 months but will eventually fade. Artificial, passive immunity is produced by extracting serum containing antibodies from an immune animal, standardizing it and injecting it into the dog which you wish to protect. Antibodies against distemper injected this way have a half life of 3 to 10 days depending upon various factors so that by 6 to 14 days the immunity is definitely below protective level.

Active immunity is produced by an invasion of antigen in a dog not previously immune. Natural infection produces an immunity if the antibody production is great enough to overcome the disease and the dog survives. This type of immunity is usually longer lasting than any other acquired immunity.

The production of immunity by artificial means is the method with which you are most familiar. This is called *vaccination*. There are six types of vaccination procedures that are used. Not all of these are used in the dog.

1. *Living organisms.*
2. *Killed organisms.*
3. *Combining living virulent organisms and immune serum.*
4. *Metabolic products.*
5. *Aggressins.*
6. *Extracts of organisms.*

I will consider them in reverse order so as to eliminate those of least importance to the dog owner. Extracts of organisms is an uncommon way of vaccinating. It is usually done using ground dried cells to get the extract.

Aggressins are used in several sheep and cattle diseases (e.g. Anthrax and Blackleg).

Metabolic products used in vaccines are those with which we are most familiar. Toxins and toxoids fall in this category. This is the method used in protecting against tetanus.

The combination of a virulent virus and an immune serum was once used to produce immunity against distemper. This was the Duncan method. It was used with great success in English countries, especially in New Zealand and Australia where, even today, the method is still employed. Its success in this country was limited, mostly because Duncan's method of serum production was not followed. With this method the dog is given both "hot" virus, which will produce the disease, and immune serum in a dose high enough to combat the virus. The result was the stimulation of antibody production, in the dog, of a very high level.

Vaccines made of killed organisms are very familiar to dog breeders. The killed vaccine is a venerable fighter against distemper and hepatitis. The infectious agent is killed either by heat or chemical and a standardized dose is injected into the dog. Several doses are used. This method is still the best method for bacterial-type vaccines such as leptospirosis, but its importance is challenged by the live vaccines now manufactured for distemper and hepatitis.

Vaccines containing living organisms are the vaccines of medical choice because it has long been recognized by most authorities that, in general, live vaccines produce the best immunity.

Some live vaccines are used in sub-lethal doses or in an abnormal area. For instance laryngotracheitis (a throat infection of poultry) vaccine is deposited in the cloaca of the chicken. This type of vaccine is not used in dogs.

Attenuated live vaccines are the common type produced for dogs. The virulent organism is grown on successive recipients abnormal for the organism until it has lost the power to produce disease, but retains the power to stimulate antibody production.

The original type was developed on chick embryo. This was the first breakthrough in modern distemper vaccination. Today the most common type utilized is a tissue-culture vaccine. Such vaccines, for hepatitis and distemper, are supported by most veterinary authorities.

Among the live vaccines we also have some heterogenous vaccines. This is a vaccine where the organism is so closely related to a second organism that it can stimulate protection against the second organism. The classic example is the protection given to humans against smallpox through the use of a cow pox organism. In dogs we have a new vaccine developed from human measles which will protect puppies from distemper at 3 weeks of age. It works on the cell level and it is not interfered with by existing antibodies nor does it interfere with later vaccines. It is thought to protect the animal up to 7 months. Its full value will have to stand the test of time. Perhaps by the time you read this we will know.

The Vaccination Program

Vaccination programs vary from area to area and veterinarian to veterinarian and I will only make general recommendations based upon known facts.

The facts we must deal with are:

1. About 85% of all puppies can be vaccinated against distemper at 9 weeks.

ADDITIVE REACTION

UNITS

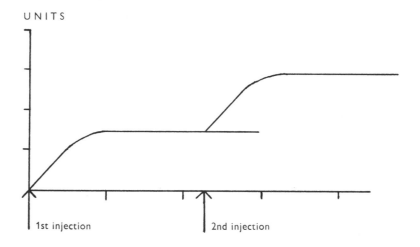

1st injection   2nd injection

AMNESTIC REACTION

UNITS

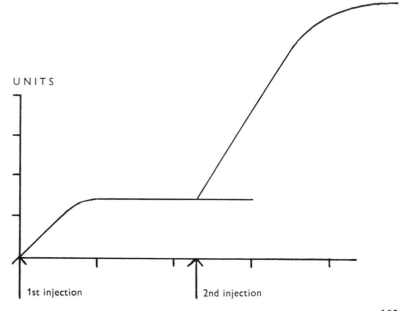

1st injection   2nd injection

2. *Under 9 weeks less than 85% become immune.*

3. *At 4 months all dogs able to utilize a vaccine can become immune against distemper.*

4. *About 2% of dogs cannot build an immunity from any vaccine.*

5. *At 3 months all dogs able to use vaccine can become immune against hepatitis.*

6. *Any globulin or serum may have an effect for up to 14 days.*

Based upon these factors it is apparent that the first vaccine should be given at about 9 weeks of age and 14 days after the last "puppy" serum shot. This may be done in one or two procedures utilizing distemper, hepatitis and leptospirosis serums. It is also apparent, for complete safety, that a follow-up distemper dose should be given as close to 4 months as possible. Thus we often have a series of vaccines.

Because it is known that the immunity conferred will wane in a third of the dogs in one year, two thirds in two years, unless infection contact ups the natural immunity, it is necessary to revaccinate with a one shot booster each year.

Many breeders now take advantage of the more scientific method of the nomograph. The nomograph is a measurement of the dam's immunity utilized to plot the best age to immunize the puppies. Based on the information gleaned from the nomograph a 95% or better take with vaccine can be realized without the trouble or expense of serum shots or the worry that the first adult vaccine may be interfered with. Any dog showing a titer of less than 100 is susceptible to distemper. Therefore, the bitch's titer is also known during the nomograph and recommendations for her for the following year can be made. Normally testing only for the purpose of finding the bitch's immunity to see if boostering is necessary is uneconomical.

Vaccine Failures

The reasons for vaccination failure vary with the vaccine used, but the greatest reason is when the vaccine falls into the hands of the layman. When purchasing a puppy supposedly "vaccinated" be sure you receive a signed veterinary certificate to that effect. If no certificate is provided check with your veterinarian before purchasing the puppy.

1. *Vaccine spoilage—This occurs with improper storage, heat, the use of out of date vaccine, premixing of vaccine, or sometimes even light exposure.*

2. *The dog is already infected with disease before vaccination.*

3. *Interference with passive antibodies from either the dam or serum renders the vaccine ineffective.*

4. *Utilizing chemicals to sterilize either the syringe or the site of vaccination on the skin of the animal may well kill live vaccines. Only disposable or heat sterilized syringes should be used.*

5. *The dog has an inherent inability to utilize vaccine to build immunity.*

Only your veterinarian can protect you from the first four failures, only luck against the fifth. The person who obtains vaccine from a non-reputable source, and this is the only source open to the layman, has no guarantee against any of the reasons for failure, your veterinarian has the guarantee of four years or more of advanced veterinary education and years more of experience.

What to Vaccinate Against

Distemper is the most important disease to protect your dog from. This dread disease is still killing or maiming better than 50% of all puppies born today. *Hepatitis* follows closely in order of seriousness and is usually incorporated in most vaccination programs.

Leptospirosis inoculation is often incorporated into the program as well. If not, it is best to request the vaccine. While the disease recovery rate is far higher than distemper or hepatitis, it nevertheless leaves permanent kidney damage which may well shorten the life of your pet.

Rabies inoculation is usually done after the dog is 6 months of age as this is the first time a lasting effect from the vaccine is ordinarily possible. Live vaccines protect for greater lengths of time than do killed. In endemic areas there are often laws requiring the vaccination be done or there may be free rabies clinics. Regardless of the possibility of your dog getting rabies in your area vaccination should be done from a public health standpoint. Protecting your dog protects you and the public against rabies (hydrophobia).

Tetanus is an uncommon disease of dogs and rarely is it necessary to vaccinate. The usual procedure is to give antitoxin when the possibility arises where tetanus becomes a threat.

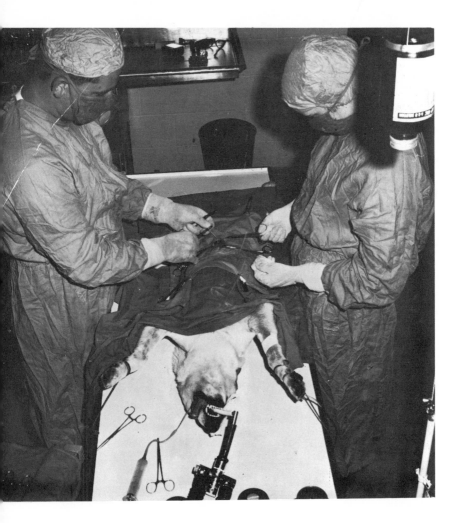

Surgical procedures in today's modern veterinary
hospitals are pursued with the same diligence and
delicate skill as similar procedures in the
finest human medical centers.

CHAPTER 8

UROGENITAL DISEASES

Diseases of the urinary system are one of the commonest afflictions of dogs over middle age. Primarily affected is the kidney. The kidney filters about 25% of the blood removing the toxic products, especially urea, and extracts the useful products. The blood is transferred via a capillary nest known as the *glomerulus*. From here the filtrate passes through a series of tubules during which water and minerals are reabsorbed. The system of tubules end in the hilus of the kidney and the urine passes down the ureters to the bladder. Infection may enter via the bloodstream or may ascend from the bladder.

Nephritis

Kidney disease—This can be acute from active sudden infection, or chronic from progressive breakdown due to past disease and overtaxing the kidney along with geriatric changes.

Interstitial nephritis is the commonest form of this disease. Here, as the course becomes more chronic, tubules are destroyed and connective tissue scars and fills up the working areas of the kidney. In the acute condition the dog may show signs of increased thirst, depression, temperature, pain in the kidney area and vomiting. Urination is usually depressed and the dog becomes dehydrated. Nephritis is often caused by leptospirosis or other bacterial infection. Urinalysis may show a high specific gravity which decreases as the disease becomes chronic. Protein is increased and blood may be present. The dog will show microscopic tubule tissue known as "casts." The BUN (blood urea nitrogen) is elevated.

In general, upon treatment, the acute cases respond well. Vomiting must be controlled and the water and electrolyte balance restored.

The latter is accomplished by intravenous drips of electrolytic fluids with sugar for energy. Vitamin B-complex is supplied the patient as these water soluble vitamins are depleted.

Antibiotics are used for infection. Penicillin-Streptomycin in combination is most used as Streptomycin is specific for Leptospirosis. Good nursing, supplying warmth and quiet, is essential. Stomach sedatives will control vomiting as oral nutrition is undertaken. The diet should be high calorie in nature. Proteins only of the highest quality (eggs, dairy products, etc.) should be used. Other protein is contraindicated. Carbohydrates may be given (oatmeal, corn syrup, toast).

Chronic interstitial nephritis is usually a condition of old dogs. *Leptospirosis* is one of the main culprits which predispose the kidneys to the disease. Here tubule loss has progressed slowly until the remaining tubules are over-taxed. The body becomes toxic and suddenly there is a kidney collapse. Uremia follows. The dog has often been unthrifty with dry coat and signs of dehydration for quite a period. There is a history of increased water intake and urination. The urine is light and resembles water. Sometimes there are periodic stomach upsets. When uremia occurs the breath smells like urea (fetid, ammonia-like). There is vomiting, temperature is normal to sub-normal accompanied by shock. The gums may have ulcers or a coating of brownish slime. The animal may be drowsy to the point of coma. Dehydration occurs rapidly. The urine is of a specific gravity between water and normal. Protein reaction is slight. Casts of cells from the kidney may be present. The BUN (amount of urea in the blood) is raised and can be followed to indicate the course of the disease.

Treatment is much the same as for the acute phase of the disease, but antibiotics are of little use except as a prophylactic against other infection attacking the weakened dog. The dog should be stabilized on a low protein diet where proteins present are of high quality and put little stress on the kidneys. Commercially prepared canned foods exist specifically for this purpose. The dog should have all the fluids he wants in order to dilute the toxic products and produce enough urine to effect this dilutionary process.

Glomerulonephritis

Here the principal lesion is in the glomerules. The condition is rare. The clinical case and treatment is much the same as for acute interstitial nephritis, except that the blood and protein are in greater amounts in the urine.

Suppurative Nephritis

Pyogenic infection of the kidney may enter via the blood or by extension. One or both kidneys may be infected. In general the signs are much the same except that pain may be greater, pus is apparent in the urine and the blood count indicates a hot infection. Antibiotics are important. Culture here may help to limit the disease more effectively if done rapidly. If an abcess occurs in one kidney only, surgical removal may be necessary.

Pyolonephritis

This is a rare disease where the pelvis or hilus of the kidney is the main target of attack. Pus and bloody urine are outstanding symptoms. Uremia may result and have to be attacked.

Nephroses

Nephroses is a primary tubule lesion. The cause may be poisons, overdosing of sulfonamides, or toxins from wounds or burns. Uremia may follow.

Treatment is as for nephritis with the removal of the offending toxin.

Kidney Stones

Although calculi (stones) may be formed in any part of the urinary tract kidney stones are uncommon. The condition is almost entirely limited to Dalmatians especially around the age of 5 years or more. This breed has the distinction of secreting uric acid like a man instead of the typical canine urea. Therefore he is prone to the formation of kidney stones like man. The dog usually shows intense pain, blood in the urine and often pus. X-ray reveals the stone. Treatment is surgical.

Less Common Kidney Conditions

Congenital cysts occur in the kidney and can cause death to the dog in early life.

Primary renal tumors are uncommon but when they do occur are usually adenocarcinomas, a type of malignant cancer. Kidneys are more commonly attacked by secondary metastatic invasion (the seeding of cancer to other areas) of a variety of types.

Dioctophyina renale is an uncommon parasite of the kidney but has the distinction of being the largest nematode worm of dogs and is therefore worthy of inclusion here.

Bladder Disease

Cystitis is an infection of the bladder. It results from either ascending or descending infections. Calculi (stones) predispose the animal to secondary infections.

The animal is distressed and indulges in frequent urination. The urine is often bloodstained. The bladder shows pain from palpation. The temperature may be raised. Unless the condition is long standing where the kidneys are toxic, uremia signs do not appear. The BUN is normal and the specific gravity is high, protein is high and blood is present. Often the urine is alkaline.

Treatment consists of antibiotics sometimes with protolytic enzymes where debris is present in excess amounts. Water should be provided in large amounts to allow flushing. Antiseptic flushes are helpful in changing the pH of the urine, especially from alkaline to acid. If tumors or calculi are present then surgery is necessary.

Bladder Stones

Urolithiasis is a condition where mineral deposits are present. These stones may be so small as to be like gravel or so large that the bladder is filled with one stone. They may be rough or smooth. If the stones are of the gravelly type, products are available which are supposed to dissolve them. The residue is then flushed into the bladder. Larger stones must be removed surgically. Recurrence is common so the dog should be put on a diet nearly ash free. Kidney diets are an excellent aid in prevention.

Urinary Incontinence

The continual dripping of urine or uncontrolled urination may be caused by several disturbances. Primary incontinence is usually a result of chronic cystitis or other bladder disease.

Any damage to the nerve control of the bladder from trauma, disc lesions, spondylitis on the spinal level, or trauma, or tumor on the central nervous system near the spinal reflex center, may cause secondary incontinence. Lesions on the sphincter muscle may also allow urine drip.

Hormones exert an influence on the autonomic nervous system and the smooth muscle of the sphincter. This explains the incontinence occurring in spayed bitches with hypoestrinism. This type is corrected with stilbestrol. Often a low maintenance dose has to be established. Congenital anatomical alterations in the ureters may also cause the condition.

The loss of bladder muscle tone (atony) is a specific bladder malfunction resulting in incontinence.

Treatment consists of clearing up the infection, emptying the bladder when control is not up to the animal and the use of cholenergic drugs which increase bladder tone.

Balanitis

This is a sheath infection of the dog. There is a constant discharge from the prepuce. This condition is usually of more bother to the owner than the dog. Antiseptic flushes usually relieve the condition.

Female Reproductive System

The bitch usually has two breeding cycles a year. Exceptions occur in Basenjis, which cycle once yearly, and Irish Setters which often cycle on an 8 month regime. Toy breeds will sometimes cycle three times in a year, especially if not bred.

The cycle has four stages:

1. *Anestrus*—This extends from the physiological end of one cycle to the beginning of another and represents a period of inactivity.

2. *Proestrus*—This stage shows the first physical signs. There is bleeding and vulvular swelling, and it usually lasts 9 days.

3. *Estrus*—This is the breeding period. It varies from 5 to 12 days but usually is of about 9 days' duration. Ovulation may occur on the second day, but seems to vary.

4. *Metestrus*—This is the stage of regressive changes. It lasts about 3 months but during the first few days the bitch often still attracts males giving the appearance of a 21 day breeding cycle. The cellular content of the discharge varies with the stage. Continuous smears will enable a veterinarian to tell when estrus is truly starting. This procedure is helpful in bitches whose breeding cycle is erratic.

The Ovary

The ovary is affected by cysts and tumors. These can cause a constant physical heat but conception does not follow. Sometimes the ovaries show juvenile degeneration and need hormonal treatment to initiate cycling. This is not always successful. With tumors or persistent cysts surgical removal may be the only answer to breeding normalcy.

Metritis

Metritis is an inflammation of the uterus. It occurs as acute, chronic, or as a pyometra.

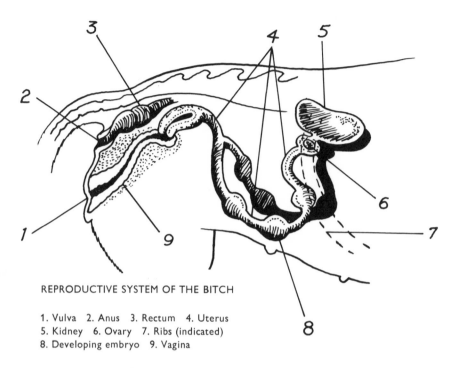

REPRODUCTIVE SYSTEM OF THE BITCH

1. Vulva   2. Anus   3. Rectum   4. Uterus
5. Kidney   6. Ovary   7. Ribs (indicated)
8. Developing embryo   9. Vagina

Acute metritis is usually the result of a contamination entering during whelping, or from retained placenta, or sometimes from ascending invaders which penetrate during a heat period. The dog shows high temperature, uterine discharge (bloody to purulent), straining, and abdominal pain. Treatment with wide range antibiotics is indicated. Often hospitalization is necessary in order to give continuous injections of pitocin to stimulate the uterus to discharge its contents. Care must be taken during pregnancy to be sure there are no puppies left in the uterus before using this drug. Indiscriminate use of pitocin can cause uterine rupture if there is a puppy stuck in the uterus and physically unable to move, regardless of the bitch's inner contractions.

If the animal is a valuable breeding bitch cultures of the discharge may be necessary to make sure the proper drug is being used. The object is to cure the infection and not just have a regressive effect on the bacteria, leaving a subclinical infection which will cause trouble in subsequent litters. Some of these cases need surgery to assure the life of the bitch.

Chronic Metritis

Chronic metritis does not always show a definite pattern. Most bitches showing poor fertility or whose puppies lack viability, will fall in this category. The bitch may show erratic cycles, lack of conception, or abortion. If puppies are born they may be dead or die shortly after birth in a typical "fading syndrome." The bitch is not usually ill but may show a mucopurulent discharge at times. The infection may be entirely subclinical showing only "fading" puppies. Successful treatment of such bitches should involve a culture and sensitivity test at a time when the cervix is open, e.g. after parturity or during a heat period. If the sample is taken at the beginning of a heat the bitch can be treated and bred with good hope of success. If the problem has been long standing it is also a good idea to re-treat during the last week of gestation to aid the possibly infected puppies as well, and perhaps just after parturition to prevent new infection. If cultures are not done antibiotics of the widest range should be used.

Congestion in the vulva
is a sign of heat. It is accompanied by
vaginal bleeding which usually
disappears a few days before
breeding time.

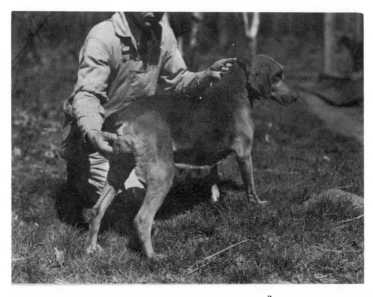

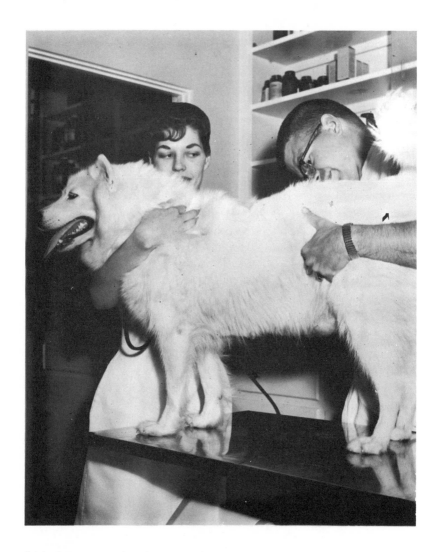

Palpitation may reveal an abnormality in the
abdominal cavity such as tumors, bladder stones,
enlarged liver, etc. Any diagnosis made in
this way will almost always need either X-ray
or laboratory tests for confirmation.

Pyometritis

This is an infection of the uterus most often seen in older and also virginal bitches. It frequently occurs a few weeks to a month following a heat period or it may be the result of an unarrested acute metritis.

The bitch first shows depression. Temperature is very high, and the vulva may emit a discharge bloody to purulent depending upon whether the uterus is open or closed. The white blood cell count is up and the abdomen may be tender. If diagnosis is in doubt, an x-ray will show the shadow of the swollen uterus.

Surgery is the only treatment for pyometritis if a successful outcome is to be expected. These cases are poor surgical risks as they can go into shock very easily. Therefore treatment for pending shock is usually indicated, high doses of antibiotics are administered and surgery is undertaken as soon as possible.

Recovery is usually rapid, considering the condition of the animal, but hospitalization is necessary for several days.

Uterine Torsion

This is a rare condition where a segment or horn of the uterus may twist. The segment may rupture and a fetus may be ejected into the abdominal cavity. Surgery is necessary.

Vaginitis

Vaginitis is seen often in the bitch puppy before the first estrus. The discharge may be sticky and grey to yellow-green. It may occur in bitches harboring Herpes virus. These cases are usually self-limiting and clear up upon the first heat.

If the discharge is copious, or if an older bitch is involved, treatment should be tried. This consists of the use of hormones and/or antibiotics both locally and systemically. This may only control the condition which may recur until a heat period is passed. The urine should be examined as vaginitis may be secondary to cystitis.

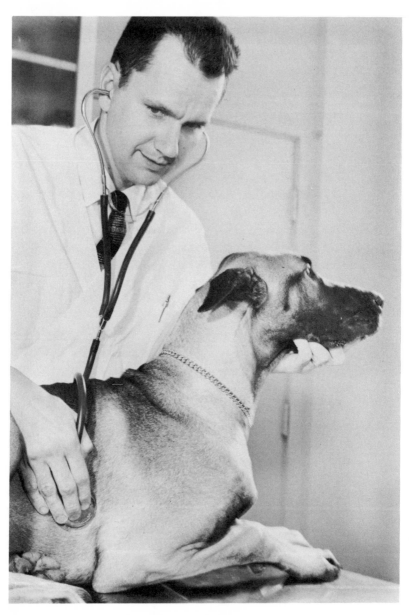

The Great Dane, with its deep and narrow thorax,
is more susceptible to respiratory infections
than many other breeds.

CHAPTER 9

RESPIRATORY DISEASES

Respiratory diseases are not as common in dogs as they are in humans probably because the dog is not susceptible to the common cold. Also there is breed variation founded upon resistance and physical structure. Hounds have a greater resistance to cold and wet than the average house dog. Breeds with deep narrow thoraxes, like Greyhounds and Great Danes, are more susceptible to and more apt to succumb to respiratory infections. Brachycephalic breeds—Bulldogs, Bostons, Boxers—have, because of their facial anatomy, a greater tendency to nasal inflammations and often have an elongated soft palate which acts as an irritating flap in the rear of the oral cavity.

It is essential to understand some basic principles in order to better appreciate the problems that accompany many respiratory conditions. First, the chest contains a negative pressure making expansion of the lungs easier. When the lungs are fully expanded the pressure is near zero, but when they deflate they remove matter from the space inside the chest producing a negative pressure. Should injury open a chest wall, the lung would collapse and be unable to inflate against normal atmospheric pressure. The dog's nasal passage is very vascular, bleeding easily from injury. Sinus in the skull bones communicates with the respiratory system. Some of these sinuses have a wall formed by the animal's teeth and thus tooth infection can lead to respiratory infection. The lungs and chest cavity are lined with pleura which is lubricated to allow free movement of the surfaces.

Air is taken into the lungs and oxygen is removed and put into the blood cells. The cells then carry the oxygen to the body tissues and return for more. Therefore, any inability of the body to get oxygen, due either to respiratory or blood problems, will cause an increase in respiration in an attempt to compensate.

Rhinitis

Rhinitis is a rare inflammation of the nasal passages. It can be caused by physical irritation or from bacterial invasion, of which Staphylococcus is the most common. Bilateral infection is most often associated with general disease but when one side only is affected it most likely is local. Remove the primary cause, such as parasites, foreign bodies or dust, and treat the infection with antibiotic nasal sprays or drops. Bleeding is treated with cold packs and quiet.

Tumors also occur in the nasal passages. The highly dangerous and malignant carcinoma is the commonest type of cancer that invades these passages. Benign polyps and "wart-like" growths occur occasionally.

(Nasal parasites are discussed under the chapter on parasites.)

Sinusitis

Sinusitis is an infection of the sinuses. The frontal sinus is in the forehead region and the maxillary is just above the rear teeth of the upper jaw.

Extension of nasal infections or tooth abcesses, or upper respiratory tract infection, can cause sinusitis.

The animal usually runs a temperature. Nasal discharge is the most common sign especially with frontal sinus infection. Occular discharge also occurs. There may be swelling around the sinus area and an open drain between the eye and the lip below in maxillary sinus infection.

Treatment is by antibiotics and often enzymes which break down pus. Surgical intervention is often necessary to establish proper drainage and the removal of infected teeth is essential.

Tonsillitis

The tonsils, which lie on the side walls of the rear of the oral cavity, commonly become inflamed. The inflammation can be the result of local area infection, part of a systemic disease such as Hepatitis, or a direct infection of the tonsils themselves.

Acute infections of the tonsils alone are bacterial and most often Streptococcus. The dog coughs, shows swelling in the neck area, vomiting and exudates at the rear of the mouth, often causing bad breath. The tonsils are enlarged and inflamed. Acute cases respond well to antibiotics.

Chronic tonsillitis is another story. The dog can show all the signs of the acute phase but usually in a milder form. Weight loss is often associated with chronic tonsillitis. When the acute condition shows poor response to treatment or the condition becomes chronic, the tonsils should be removed.

Great Danes seem to be particularly prone to tonsillitis and their response to drug therapy is poor. In the author's hospital it is usually recommended that a tonsillectomy be performed on this breed when the condition is found.

Tonsils are also a common site for tumors. More often than not these growths are found to be malignant.

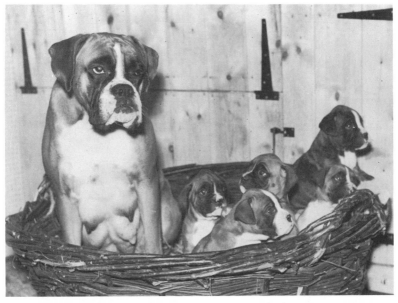

Boxers and other brachycephalic breeds are prone to nasal infection.

Laryngitis

While infection extending from the surrounding areas can cause inflammation of the larynx, the most common cause of laryngitis is from excessive barking.

Tracheobronchitis

Tracheobronchitis is an inflamation of the trachea (the wind pipe) and the bronchii. While this infection can be a part of general respiratory disease, it is usually a specific infection of the area and is often referred to as "kennel cough." The condition is highly contagious and any dogs confined with a "kennel cough" dog are very apt to get this aggravating disease.

Many agents have been named as the causative factor but as yet the problem has not been resolved. At the present moment it is thought that virus is the most likely cause complicated by a "PPLO" organism and, often, *Brucella bronchiseptica* bacteria.

The disease is very aggravating but not dangerous as far as mortality is concerned.

The dog has a dry hacking cough that is persistent. But the dog is usually bright, exhibits good appetite and is apparently normal otherwise. The course of the disease may be several weeks in length but eventually is self limiting.

Very wide-range antibiotics, sulfonamides and cough suppressants, are used to treat the condition.

Chronic Bronchitis

This is a chronic inflammation of the bronchial tube. While it can be primary, it usually results as a secondary condition from previous respiratory, heart, or oral infections. Chemicals, dust and smoke can cause the primary irritation. The resulting condition is an inflammation which is characterized by a chronic productive cough. The dog usually loses condition and may cough for months or years. Temperature is usually normal but the dog is susceptible to secondary infection.

The condition is usually incurable due to chronic scarring of the bronchials but the cough can be suppressed with cough medication, especially at night to allow peaceful sleep. Care must also be taken to see that the general health and condition of the dog is kept up to par.

Bronchiectasis

Bronchiectasis is the abnormal dilation of the bronchials. The breakdown of the living cells causes saccules which gather exudates. Symptomatically, the dog shows a chronic productive cough accompanied by a fetid, purulent discharge. The condition may be months or years old. It can be acquired either for an unknown, spontaneous reason, or as a result of respiratory infection, or it may be congenital.

During bad attacks the dog may show signs of pneumonia with

temperature rise. Chest noises increase (not in bronchitis). Diagnosis is based on clinical symptoms, history and x-rays which show bronchial dilation and sacculation.

Treatment is based on keeping the canine patient in general health. Cough suppressants are not used as the fetid mucus must be gotten up. Antibiotics are reserved for attacks during which the animal's temperature rises.

Parasitic Bronchitis. (See parasites, *Filaroides osleri*)

Pulmonary Catastrophies

Pulmonary fibrosis occurs as a result of chronic respiratory disease and causes the fibrotic scarring and destruction of parts of the lung.

Pulmonary edema is a filling of part of the lung with exudates until air cannot enter the lung. It occurs as part of pneumonia with certain allergic reactions, or is secondary to cardiac disease. Treatment is directed at relieving the underlying cause.

Atelectasis is collapse of the lung due to obstruction from parasites, tumors, exudates or hydrothorax. Treatment consists of removing the underlying cause and the use of antibiotics to prevent infection.

Emphysema is rupture within the lungs which fills with air. It occurs with the onslaught of respiratory disease or from senile changes. It is not very important as it seldom spreads far.

Pneumonia

Pneumonia is an infection of the lungs that takes many forms.

Interstitial pneumonia involves the total living tissue and is usually viral in nature.

Almost all cases are the pneumonic part of distemper. Treatment is as for distemper.

Lobar pneumonia, or *bronchopneumonia*, involves a lobe of the lung and is usually bacterial and secondary to viral pneumonia. There is mucus, pus and blood in the lung (not in interstitial). Occular purulent discharge is also present.

Aspiration pneumonia is caused by the breathing in of fluids, vomit and medications.

Verminous pneumonia is caused by a parasitic invasion of the lungs during hook and round worm migration. The eosinophils of the white blood cells rise and secondary bacterial invasion may occur.

Hypostatic pneumonia is common only in old dogs. It occurs in dogs unable to move about which results in a migration of fluids and exudates to one area of the lung. Bacteria grow fast and well in such a medium.

Mycotic pneumonia is a fungus pneumonia. Various fungi or yeasts can cause this type of pneumonia.

General symptoms of pneumonia are mainly a difficulty in breathing and shortness of breath. Breathing may be abdominal in nature due to the dog being unwilling because of pain to move the chest walls. The stethescope discloses abnormal lung sounds.

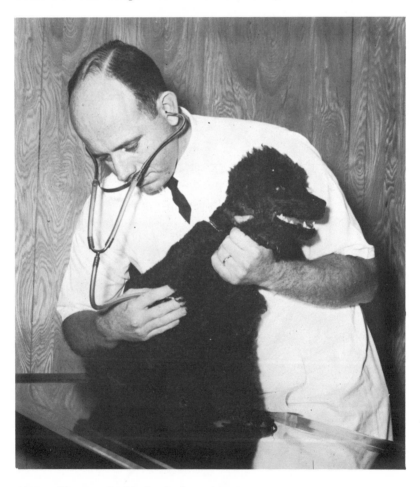

Abnormal lung sounds picked up by the stethescope can indicate mycotic pneumonia, a fungal respiratory disease. Other symptoms include shortness of breath and difficulty in breathing.

Treatment is with antibiotics, general nursing and attacking any general underlying cause (parasites, distemper, etc.). The fungal type may respond to the newer fungicides.

Pleura

Pleurisy is either dry or wet and most often associated with, or predisposing to pneumonia. In wet pleurisy the cavity fills with pus blocking lung sounds and leaving no area for lung expansion. Dry pleurisy discloses dry friction sounds. Pain is the outstanding sign. Temperature is usually high. Pleurisy is usually a symptom of some other disease so the underlying cause should be found and treated.

Pneumothorax

Pneumothorax is the accumulation of air in the pleural cavity. It is usually caused by an injury in the chest wall and often results in the collapse of a lung. Air must be removed and usually the rent repaired.

Diaphragmatic Hernia

Hernia of the diaphragm occurs almost always as the result of trauma, especially auto accidents. The diaphram is a wall of muscle between the abdominal cavity and the thorax. Surgical repair is necessary.

Neoplasms

Cancer of the lungs is common but more often of secondary metastatic nature rather than primary tumor.

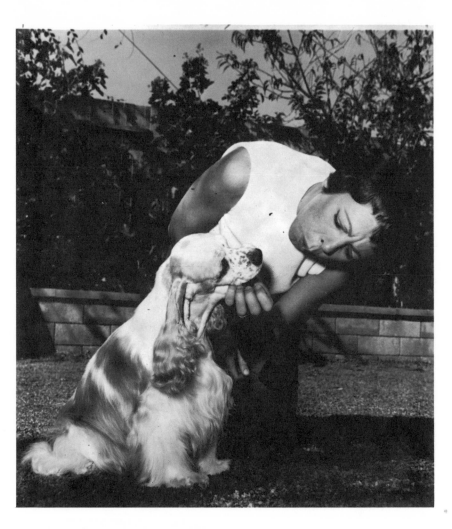

Cocker Spaniels are prone to infection of the lip
fold, as are many other deep-lipped breeds. But it
is so common in Cockers that
it is referred to as "Cocker Mouth."
Treatment is with antibiotics locally and
generally, but sometimes surgery is indicated.

CHAPTER 10

ALIMENTARY TRACT DISEASES

Diseases of the alimentary tract are the most common complaints of dogs. Care must be taken in diagnosis to ascertain whether the complaint is regional or a reflection of disease outside the tract (e.g. distemper).

The Lips

Infection of the lips is usually an extension of infection elsewhere on the body that the dog has been orally keeping clean by licking. Pustules, rawness and suppuration are common. Treatment is with antibiotics locally and generally.

Infection in the lip fold along the sides of the face is common especially in long-lipped dogs. It is so common in Cocker Spaniels that it is referred to as a "Cocker Mouth." Treatment is as above but at times the surgical removal of the fold is both indicated and easier.

Stomatitis

Stomatitis is an infection of the mouth. It is commonly caused by foreign bodies, hot foods, chemicals, or extension infections from tonsils, teeth, etc. Stomatitis also occurs in vitamin B deficiency.

Candida albicans, a fungus, causes a mycotic stomatitis.

Treatment is directed at removing the cause and the use of antibiotics to halt the infection. Antiseptic solutions, especially with mycotic stomatitis, are also used.

Infectious Oral Papillomatosis

There is a benign wart growth which can occur, usually in the mouth of puppies. It is viral in nature. The growths cause irritation, difficulty in eating, and may even hinder breathing, but not generally. The condition is irritating but not serious. The growths should be left alone as removal may cause a spreading of the condition. There is a spontaneous normal recovery within 3 weeks. Specific vaccine is available but its usefulness is difficult to determine because it takes about as long to work as the self-cure takes.

Teeth

Enamel Erosion

Although erosion can be caused by chemicals, enzymes or bacteria, the cause, in more than 99% of the cases, is due to distemper contracted by the patient at an early age.

Retained Baby Teeth

Retained baby teeth is a common problem in small breeds. Most will fall out at 7 or 8 months of age but if they persist they should be pulled or they may cause deviations in the adult teeth.

Tartar

Tartar formation is the most prevalent tooth problem of our pets, since they are not susceptible to cavities. Dogs are kept on soft diets which is normal for household pets but which promotes tartar development so that dogs over 5 years of age often need dental cleaning. Toy breeds are more susceptible than larger breeds to tartar formation. Some authorities recommend giving bones and hard foods to promote tooth cleaning through scraping action, but I rather lean away from this solution of the problem except with very large bones that the animals are unable to break up and swallow. I feel that dental work two or three times in a dog's lifetime is not a burden on the owner who demands a life-time of love and companionship from the dog, and I much prefer cleaning teeth to removing pieces of bone from the intestinal tract at 3 A.M. or giving enemas to dogs unable to pass masses of bone chips in their stool.

The Gums

The gums are subject to local and extension infection. They react to chronic disease and vitamin deficiencies. Poisoning with heavy metals, such as lead, causes a blue line along the gums, and bleeding.

Treatment is aimed at correcting the initiating cause and the use of antiseptics or antibiotics to clear infection.

Certain brachycephalic breeds, especially Boxers, are subject to a multiple benign growth of the gums. This is best removed surgically, cauterization being the most common method. If not treated the dog will develop difficulty in eating.

The Tongue

Inflammation of the tongue is known as *Glossitis* and is caused by insect stings, lack of blood supply, chemical burns, and as an accompanying part of leptospirosis or distemper. (See treatment for the specific listed causes.)

Salivary Glands

These are rarely infected but they may develop cysts from a blocked duct. Surgical removal is recommended.

The Pharynx

Since this area at the back of the oral cavity links with both the respiratory and the alimentary tract it is affected by extensions of infections of both systems to cause a "sore throat."

Esophagitis

The *esophagus* can be irritated by chemicals or infection, but its

House pets on soft diets need dental care more frequently than dogs provided with some hard foods. Tartar should not be allowed to accumulate.

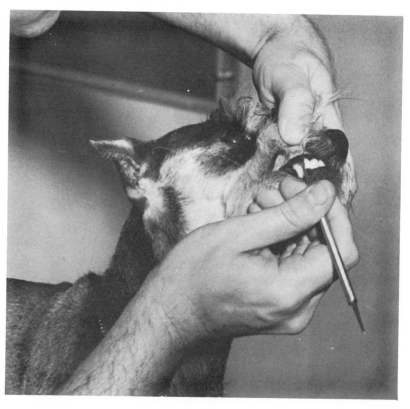

most common problems are congenital dilation and dilation and blockage associated with persistent right aortic arch of the heart. These problems are discussed under pediatrics.

The Stomach

Acute Gastritis—Acute Gastritis can have many causes and is characterized by sudden persistent vomiting and abdominal pain.

Overheating, allergy to food, bad food, foreign bodies, chemicals and irritating medications (often the licking of skin medications) are the common dietary problems causing gastritis. It can also be caused by infection from bacteria, from general disease or parasitic disease. It is necessary to try to find and assess the primary cause, from the patient's clinical history, and remove it or to treat the general disease.

Antiemetics and antibiotics are often used in combination. Erythymycin and Neomycin are excellent oral antibiotics for gastro-intestinal problems as they are not absorbed by the gut.

Diet should be liquid and bland during the first few days. Add solids to the bland diet slowly, and after several more days return gradually to the feeding of the normal diet.

Chronic Gastritis

Chronic gastritis occurs when there has been disturbed digestive and functional changes to the gastric wall over a period of time. Repeated attacks of acute gastritis and foreign bodies are the most common causes. Stricture at the end of the stomach, limiting the amount of food allowed out, also causes chronic gastritis. Lastly chronic toxic conditions such as kidney disorders, cause chronic gastric changes.

One of the author's first surgical cases was a chronic gastritis due to a foreign body. It seems that in Australia there is a belief that copper prevents distemper. Many people believing in this fable wrap copper wire around the dog's collar. My erstwhile client went them one better and fed his dog two large copper Australian pennies. The removal of the pennies, the chronic gastritis, and the eventual cost reformed this worthy person so that he never wanted "to get his tuppence worth" in again!

Chronic gastritis is treated by removing the cause, controlling the vomiting and using a bland diet while stimulating the gastric juices with drugs.

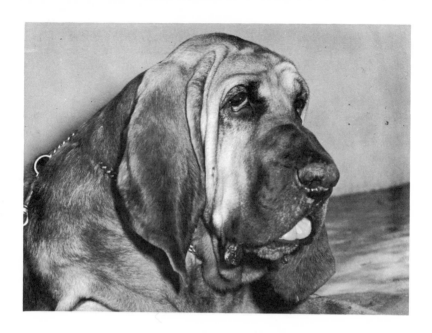

Bloodhounds, Saint Bernards, and Great Danes
have a definite predisposition to the
condition known as bloat.

Bloat (*Gastric dilation and/or torsion*)

Bloat is a gastric dilation of the stomach often accompanied by a 90° to 180° twisting of the stomach so as to lock off the ends.

Bloodhounds, Great Danes, and Saint Bernards have a definite predisposition to the condition. Other large breeds are more apt to be victims than small breeds.

The onset is sudden. The abdomen is grossly distended and respiration hampered and short. Dilation is so rapid in some dogs that one can actually discern the growth. The dog may attempt unsuccessfully to vomit. Tapping on the distension produces a tympanic sound.

Some authorities say that certain diets and times of eating will help to prevent the condition, but in the author's experience with prominent Bloodhound and Dane kennels, no changes in diet or time lessened or changed the incidence of the disease. Diagnosis is on clinical examination. It remains only to decide if a twist is present or not.

Passage of a stomach tube is sometimes possible in simple dilation. When it is determined by the veterinarian that there is no twist, certain drugs and stomach tubing will often relieve the condition. But if it cannot be immediately determined, emergency surgery to relieve the gas and replace the stomach in its proper position must be done. Intravenous drips to prevent the almost inevitable accompanying shock should be started. Recent information indicates the use of calcium IV as an adjunctive treatment. While this is yet to be proved anything that might help, and that will definitely not harm, should be done.

The prognosis is very grave with a very high rate of mortality. The earlier the condition is discovered and treatment undertaken the better are the chances of success.

Pyloric Spasm

This is a spasm of the muscles at the end of the stomach usually associated with nervous dogs of the brachycephalic type. There is chronic vomiting usually associated with excitement. The condi-

The muscles at the end of a dog's stomach
can go into spasm resulting in what is called
pyloric spasm. Boston Terriers sometimes exhibit it.

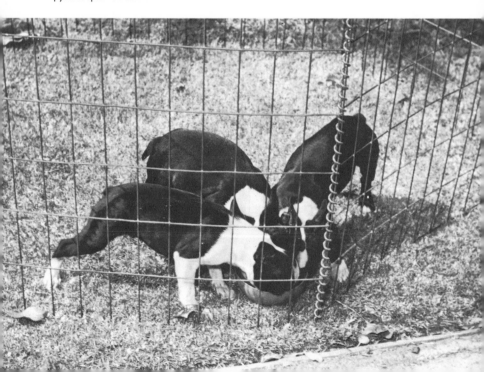

tion is very long-standing. The use of tranquilizers will help to relieve the condition but surgical repair is the only path to a full cure.

Intestines

Intestinal upsets (*enteritis*) with diarrhea and sometimes vomiting are very common, and often require laboratory work, clinical work, x-ray, or even exploratory surgery to reach full diagnosis. These upsets have varied patterns from acute to chronic. Fortunately the majority of these intestine conditions are simple inflammations which respond to generalized treatment.

Such upsets often involve the entire intestinal tract and, as often as not, the stomach, too. They will be discussed in reference to their causes, but it should be remembered that almost all have a few basic symptoms: diarrhea with or without blood, and abdominal pain often accompanied by vomiting.

Parasites are one of the easiest causes to recognize. Fecal examination to locate the eggs and response to treatment will sort out the problem. Hookworm and whipworm are the most common causes in adults, while round worm and hookworm are more common in puppies.

Bacteria or their toxins are the most common cause. This happens most frequently during the winter months, especially when warm spells occur. Often the stools are blood-stained and the dog has some fever, appetite may or may not be affected. *Streptococcus, Staphylococcus, Salmonella* and *Proteus* are the common bacteria involved. If the dog does not respond to general intestinal antibiotic therapy and bowel tighteners, cultures of the stool must be made so that the bacteria and its sensitivity can be pinpointed.

Spirochetal diarrhea has been seen but it is uncommon. It usually responds to the same general antibiotic treatment used in bacterial fostered intestinal upsets.

Protozoa can be a significant problem. Coccidiosis is discussed under parasites and it is perhaps the most common of the protozoans especially in puppies. Giardia, Trichomonas, Balantidium and Entamoeba species also occur. With careful study the protozoa can be found with fecal smears. Special anti-protozoal drugs are used and give good response.

Chemicals such as topical medications used for skin conditions, heavy metals (e.g. arsenic, phosphorus) and phenol compounds are a few of the chemical causes. The cause should be removed. An antidote is administered where possible or the dog is made to vomit or given an enema if ingestion is only a few hours old. Usually, by the time it is diagnosed, the case has progressed to the degree that stomach and intestinal sedatives, and liners such as kaopectate, are the most helpful medication during the period it takes for the chemicals to wear off.

Food allergies are also a possibility. If suspected, the food should be changed and results scrutinized carefully. Skin tests for food allergies are still embryonic in dogs so are not usually helpful. Shellfish, eggs, and horse meat, are common offenders.

Foreign bodies, especially sharp ones, often cause acute problems and are linked with much pain. They can usually be identified with x-ray. While most will eventually pass, enemas may help. In some cases surgery is necessary.

Generalized disease is the most dangerous cause as we must be sure to recognize the main disease. Diarrhea can be a sign in distemper, hepatitis and leptospirosis. Here treatment is directed at symptomatic relief and treating the main disease.

There are a few basic principles in treating diarrhea. Diets should be adjusted. In severe cases all food may be withheld and the dog given intravenous feedings of balanced electrolytes. Diets prescribed are usually bland and non-bulky. There are some special prescription diets available that are excellent. At times boiled rice and hamburger are recommended, particularly if the cause is only environmental or due to a change in diet. General stomach and intestinal liners and sedatives are good adjunctive treatment. Kaopectate and like compounds are excellent. Often these contain an antibiotic. Atropine and like drugs slow the intestinal motility. Antibiotics are commonly employed, especially neomycin, streptomycin and certain of the sulfonamides. Remember, that proper diagnosis with selective use of the above medications is essential so leave the treatment of diarrhea in the experienced hands of your veterinarian.

Constipation

When the dog is unable to pass his stool he is constipated. Any stool that is forced out is usually hard and dry and accompanied by pain. More often than not the fault is with the owner and is caused by neglect or ignorance of canine dietary needs. Bones are the most common cause. Dogs and bones do not go together—except to the veterinarian for an enema. Long-haired breeds which are not groomed often lick and swallow enough hair to cause a bowel blockage. The feeding of dry bulky foods without enough water is another owner-induced cause. Constipation also occurs with prostatic enlargement, blocking tumors, and anal gland infection. Old dogs may become constipated due to a loss of elasticity in the bowel.

The animal shows pain, enlarged abdomen, has not defecated in some time, and may be vomiting. Rectal examination or x-ray will reveal the fecal mass.

Mineral oil is good in early cases or where blockage is not complete. Most often an enema is necessary. Sometimes only surgery will relieve the condition.

Prevention lies mainly in owner education, grooming, and attention to the anal glands. When there is a lack of bowel tone, diets should be bland and non-bulky. Mineral oil or other lubricants are used prophylactily. Olive oils and other feeding oils are not very good as the dog utilizes these as sustenance. Mineral oil and paraffin will pass through and aid in lubrication.

Obstruction

Obstruction may be from a foreign body such as a golf ball, peach pit, etc. or from an intestinal calamity. Intersuseption occurs when the intestine telescopes into itself; twisting of the bowel and hernias such as umbilical hernias that may strangulate a loop of bowel are common calamities. Tumors and even enteritis can cause obstruction.

If the obstruction is high in the tract, symptoms of pain, vomiting upon eating, and shock are acute, and immediate treatment is necessary. If the blockage is lower down, the symptoms are milder. Vomiting may be unrelated to food and the dog may become toxic over a period of days.

Surgical removal of the offender is almost always the treatment, especially in high blockage. Treating enteritis and enemas may help in low blockages or infections.

Anal Glands

The dog has two glands near the anal opening similar in location to the familiar scent glands of a skunk. They have little use in the dog. They lubricate the feces when it is passed and discharge a smelly substance during fright but are for the most part vestigial and non-essential for the dog.

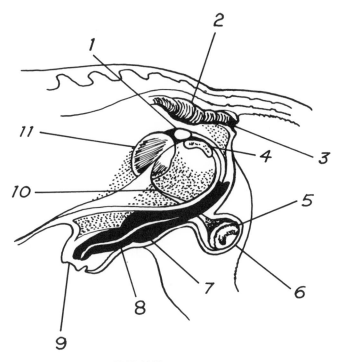

DIAGRAM OF MALE REPRODUCTIVE AND
ANAL SYSTEM

1. Prostate   2. Rectum   3. Site of anal glands
4. Section of pelvic bone   5. Testicle
6. Scrotum   7. Bulb (section of penis)
8. Peni   9. Sheath   10. Vas deferens   11. Bladder

The glands may become infected and rupture, or impacted and rupture, or they can become neoplastic.

They should be emptied when infected or impacted. This emptying is a normal grooming procedure. Antibiotics can be infused for infection.

When ruptured they should be removed (a bloody surgery) or simply burned out with electric or chemical cauterization.

Neoplasms require surgery, often extensive, because malignancy is common.

The Liver

All inflammations of the liver are called hepatitis. *Infectious Hepatitis* is a special viral condition (see infectious diseases—viral). It is

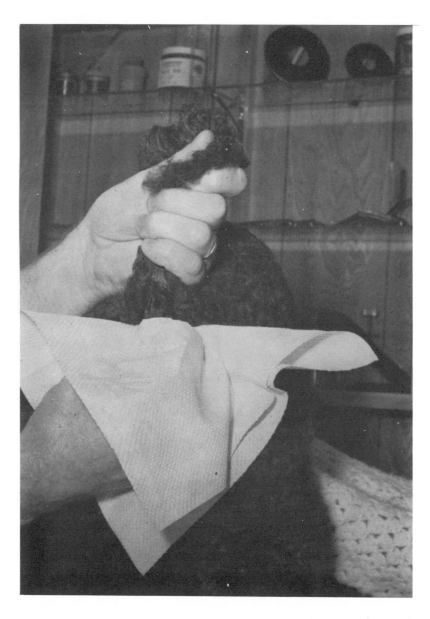

The anal glands may become enlarged and
infected if they are not naturally discharged.
If they become neoplastic from lack of attention,
surgery will be required. To prevent
infection, they should be manually emptied
during grooming.

involved in almost all normal body processes essential to the body. It helps in digestion with the bile from the gall bladder, detoxifies substances, is involved in metabolism, receives and filters the blood returning to the body and deposits many body needs such as phagocytes and glucogen. There are many liver function tests available. Most of these tests are difficult and require extensive laboratory facilities.

The liver has tremendous powers of recuperation and reserve; 80% of the liver can be diseased and the stricken animal can still survive.

Chemicals such as arsenic, phosphorus, tetrachlorethylene (a common wormer) cause toxic hepatitis when present in excess. A yellow atrophy occurs which is probably a toxic condition.

Cirrhosis, which is liver cell degeneration replaced by fibrous tissue, is caused by constant attacks on the liver by disease, toxins, parasites, low protein diet, and malnutrition.

Fatty degeneration occurs with diabetes mellitus and pancreatic disease. Congestion occurs with blood back-up especially with cardiac disease.

General symptoms are digestive upsets with vomiting, often bile-stained, tucked up appearance, palpably enlarged liver, and pain in the liver area. Ascites (fluid in the abdominal cavity) is sometimes found as well as jaundice.

Treatment consists of relieving the primary cause, e.g. treating diabetes, viral hepatitis, removing toxic substances. Diets should be regulated to take the strain off the liver. Salts should be restricted, fats should be very low. Eggs, meat, cottage cheese and skimmed milk are excellent. Prescription protein diets are very good as they are low in fat and bulk but high in protein. Diuretics help remove fluid. Choline and methionine with liver extract helps the liver digest food, especially fats.

Pancreas

The *pancreas* is a gland which secretes many digestive juices. Pancreatitis is very painful and can cause sudden death in the acute form and cause gradually debilitating disease in the chronic form.

Acute pancreatitis is characterized by severe abdominal pain, vomiting, increased heart rate, thirst and diarrhea. The dog goes rapidly into shock. Any stools passed are incompletely digested and fatty.

Treatment is first for shock with intravenous drips and corticosteroids. Antibiotics will stop infection or prevent secondary infection. Follow-up treatment is the same as recommended for chronic pancreatitis.

Chronic pancreatitis is characterized by a loss of weight while a ravenous appetite is present, fecal changes (usually smelly, greyish, putty-like with excess fat) and some abdominal pain, usually intermittent with recurring attacks. The animal may eat its own stools.

Diagnosis is suspected on clinical signs and confirmed by laboratory tests for the presence of pancreatic juices in the stool.

Treatment is achieved through the replacement of pancreatic enzymes with synthetic products, a low fat diet and choline for fat digestion.

Peritoneum

The *peritoneum* is the lining of the abdominal cavity. It also reflects on the organs. It becomes infected from extension, infections of other organs, punctures with contaminated objects, and contamination from degenerating blocked bowel. Peritonitis is painful and dangerous. Temperature is raised. Treatment is with antibiotics to control and eliminate the specific infection.

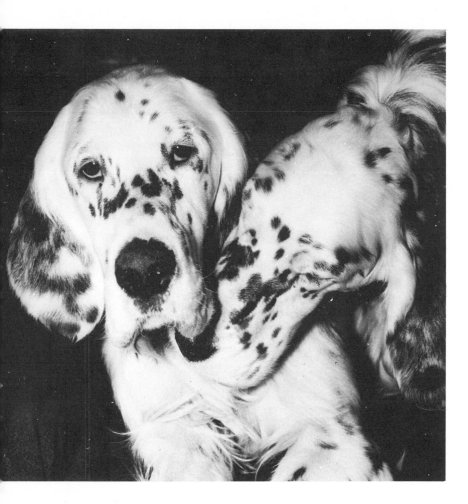

Hemophilia appears in dogs as well as humans.
It is a genetic (recessive) blood clotting deficiency
disease that is carried by the
female but exhibited by the male. The
disease cannot be cured, but a
special drug can be utilized to slow
the dissolving of healing blood clots.

CHAPTER 11

DISEASES OF THE HEART, BLOOD, AND LYMPH SYSTEMS

Congestive Heart Failure

Congestive heart failure is the most common heart disease of dogs. Coronaries as seen in man are rarely, if ever, encountered in dogs but congestive heart failure is a common condition of dogs over 6 years of age.

The basic defects causing the heart condition can be old congenital defects such as a stenosis or "hole in the heart" (as discussed under pediatrics), or the cause may be acquired. Warty growths on the valves, or heart muscle disease, are acquired often as a result of bacterial infection elsewhere in the body migrating to this site. Heart worm and tumors cause physical blocking and narrowing of the valvular areas of the chambers of the heart thus bringing on the disease.

Physically the heart defect causes a backward or forward problem. The backward problem is that this important organ is unable to pump out the blood delivered to it from the venous system thus causing a back-up and pressure on the systems of the heart, lungs, and the veins behind the heart, resulting in congestion. The increase in back pressure has an effect even on the kidney function. The forward problem is one of reduced heart output which results in arterial changes, and also causes kidney functional disturbances.

Blood enters the right side of the four chambered heart (2 chambers right and 2 chambers left). It passes from the great veins to the right atrium, to the right ventricle to the lungs, to the left atrium, to the left ventricle, and out to the arteries. The four chambers have valves between them and between the ventricles and their receivers (Pulmonary and aortic valves). Defects in the valvular regions, or in the chambers or heart muscle, can cause heart failure. Dogs with right side heart failure tire easily, and often show cyonosis, due to lack of blood reaching the lungs where needed for extra oxygen carrying. The pressure backs up, enlarging and damaging the liver. This may result in fluids in the abdominal cavity (*acites*) and subcutaneous fluid swelling (*edema*). With left failure, the pressure forcing backward causes lung congestion, this in turn brings pressure upon the right side. There may be a heart cough due to the stress upon the lungs.

Chest fluids and kidney stress, may eventually occur in conjunction with heart failure.

Treatment is directed at the side effects as well as the heart. Digitalis is used to slow the heart and increase the force and efficiency of the pumping action. Diuretics are used to remove excess body fluids. Bronchial dialators, antihistamines and other cough repressants are useful. Salt intake is lowered and the diet is adjusted to relieve the strain on the liver. Rest is important while the condition is brought under control.

Other Heart Conditions

Premature ventricular beats may exist due to overdosing with digitalis. They also occur with congestive heart failure and then are

Typical clinical picture of a dog with congestive heart failure. The animal visually exhibits ascites, or fluid in the abdominal cavity, and edema, or fluids in tissues under the neck and in the hind legs.

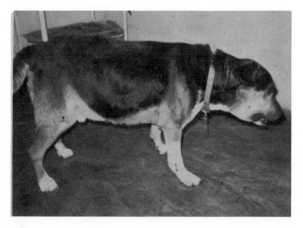

treated with digitalis and general congestive failure procedures.

Heart block is the inability of one part of the heart to send stimulation to another part of the heart. Usually treatment is unsuccessful.

Atrial fibrilation is an irregular rhythm in the atrium. It is treated with digitalis.

Pericardial effusion is the filling of the sac enclosing the heart with fluids. Surgical drainage is necessary.

Congenital heart diseases are discussed in the Chapter on pediatrics, and heart worm under parasites.

Thrombosis

Thrombosis is a mass of platelets, fibrin and cellular elements of the blood. An embolism is a small mass that breaks loose and lodges in and blocks a blood vessel.

Thrombosis in dogs usually results from local venous infection. Emboli may block the pulmonaries causing sudden death or pulmonary distress, or may block a major vessel causing a disappearance of pulse below it. Death of tissue and malfunction commonly follow emboli.

Arteriosclerosis

A rare disease in dogs which usually causes no clinical problems.

Blood Clotting Diseases

Hemorrhage may be due to direct injury of the vessels or due to infection (Hepatitis and Leptospirosis) or allergy effects upon the permeability of blood vessels. It can also be due to abnormalities in the blood such as platelet damage from chemicals or disease, hemophilia, dicumarol poisoning, vitamin K deficiency, or defects that cause the breakdown of clots (fibrinolysis).

Treatment is directed at removing the cause or correcting the defect and replacing the blood, either quickly during great loss, via transfusion, or with the use of B_{12} and Iron for long term therapy. Injuries are treated by tying off the offending vessels where necessary or practical and applying cold and pressure to the area. Coagulating drugs are often employed. Often transfusions are needed, especially following accident cases that are accompanied by shock and hemorrhage.

The basic disease is the first site of treatment, whether it involves the vessels or the platelets. Platelet defects often occur with spleen disease (the spleen must be removed surgically), leukemia diseases (terminal), or with the disease purphra, a hypersensitivity condition which occurs only rarely and usually following other disease (Corticosteroids are used for purphra). In dicumarol poisoning (a rat poison), vitamin K is replaced in the clotting formula and the clotting reaction is stopped. Vitamin K deficiency causes a parallel problem. Treatment is the administration of vitamin K.

True Hemophilia is a genetic (recessive) blood clotting deficiency disease carried by the female and exhibited by the male. The disease is incurable.

With fibrinolysis a drug, Amicar, is used to slow down the dissolving of the clot.

Autoimmune Hemolytic Anemia

This is a specific type of anemia that causes the dog to produce antibodies against its own blood cells, thus causing a short blood

Dogs do not have inherent antibodies against alien blood types as do humans. Therefore, though Type A-negative is the universal donor in dogs, most animals can accept one transfusion from an unknown donor.

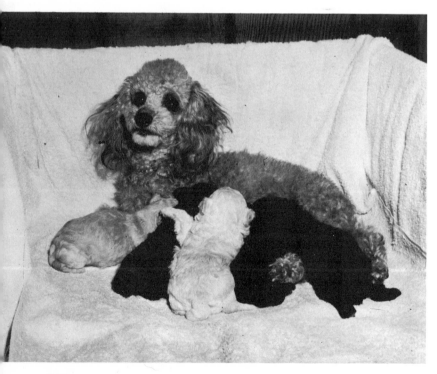

cell life and, therefore, anemia. Corticosteroids are used for treatment while blood transfusions, often contraindicated, are reserved only for emergency use.

Anemia

Anemia is the reduction of hemoglobin per unit of blood. Hemoglobin is the blood pigment which carries oxygen to the body tissues. The reduction of hemoglobin may be due to a reduction in the number of red blood cells, reduction in the size of the red blood cell, or in the amount of hemoglobin in the cell. Anemia is not in itself a disease but a sign of disease.

Anemia can be caused by blood loss. Acute blood loss is from a vessel or organ (especially spleen or liver) rupture or damage, or from a coagulation defect. Shock occurs rapidly but upon correction of the loss, and often with replacement transfusion, recovery is rapid and the body replaces the blood with stepped-up production. While Type A-negative is the universal donor in dogs, most dogs can accept one transfusion from an unknown donor until sensitized by the first transfusion, since they do not have inherent antibodies against other alien types such as humans do. Chronic blood loss is more insidious. The dog can adjust to a greater loss over a longer period without shock. Chronic loss is caused by bladder hemorrhage associated with bladder stones, hookworm, and other worm infections. Chronic bowel infection, or ulcers, or any other chronic condition causing vessel permeability also causes chronic blood loss. Treatment is directed at removing the cause, transfusions if necessary, and general deficiency anemia treatments, a subject which will be considered a bit later.

A second grouping of anemias is due to a disturbance in the blood building system. Vitamin B complex deficiencies and sometimes Vitamin C, amino acid, and protein and iron deficiencies are the causes of most of the deficiency anemias. Replacement of the lacking vitamins, proteins or minerals is the basic medical attack to promote normalcy.

Other than total blood loss hookworm also causes an iron deficiency affecting blood production. Certain infections, especially chronic infections such as metritises, cause an effect on the blood building systems, as do neoplasms (cancer).

Aplastic anemia is also a blood production defect caused by reduced bone marrow activity due to the action of toxic substances

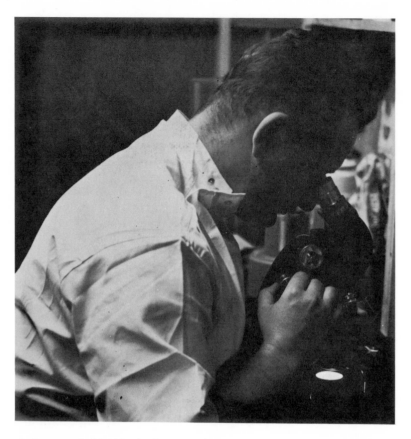

An increase of white blood cells, especially
juvenile cells, is common in human leukemia,
but is not usually found in
canine leukemia except, perhaps, terminally.

such as heavy metals, radiation, infections, and leukemia.

Lastly, anemia is caused by the destruction of blood cells. Protozoans such as Babesia directly attack the blood cell as do the toxins
of some bacteria (*Clostridium welchii* and some streptococci). Lead
and naphthalene poisoning produces a chemical attack on the blood
cells. Incompatible transfusions cause cell destruction. This type of
anemia also follows when extensive areas of the body have been
badly burned.

In all anemias the primary attack is on the causative agent with
adjunctive treatment of Vitamin B complex, Vitamin B_{12}, iron and
high protein.

The White Blood Cells

The white blood cells are the protective cells of the body. Changes in these cells indicate the presence of infection. A leukopemia or decrease of white blood cells occurs in viral disease, destruction of blood, cancer with bone marrow destruction, or with the channeling of white cells to other tissues when needed.

Leukocytosis, or an increase of white cells, is a common reaction to disease stress, though different cells react in varied ways.

Bacterial infection causes an increase especially in neutorphils, but as the condition becomes chronic the lymphocytes show a greater increase. Monocytes increase in diseases such as tuberculosis and Nocardiosis. Eosinophils increase in allergy reaction, eosinophilic myocitis and adrenal cortical disease. While a great increase of white blood cells is common in human leukemia, especially juvenile cells, it is an uncommon finding in canine leukemia except, perhaps, terminally.

Malignant Lymphoma

Malignant lymphoma is the common dog leukemia. The dog first shows swelling of the lymph nodes in the neck under the jaw. Soon other lymph nodes swell, often at the shoulder and in the inguinal region between the thigh and the body, as well as in the thigh itself. The dog becomes listless, weak, loses appetite and sometimes has difficulty breathing. As the condition progresses the dog becomes thin, experiences vomiting and is anemic. The blood picture is not diagnostic early in the disease as with humans but there may be a white cell rise late in the disease. A biopsy is the method of choice for confirmation of the disease. The condition is terminal in from 3 to 6 months.

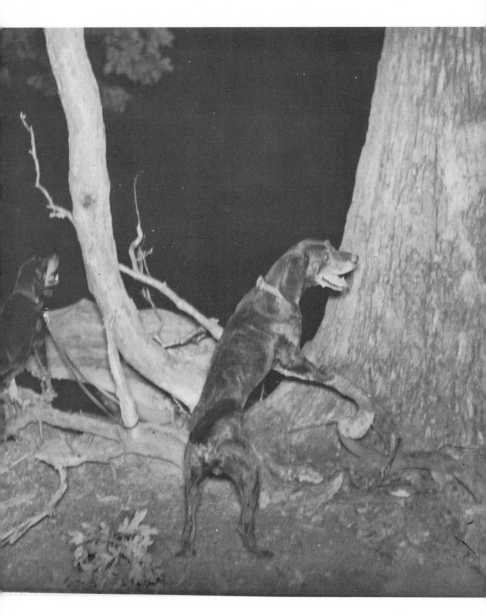

Coon Hound paralysis is a neuritis of unknown
cause. It is generally associated with
Coon Hounds simply because it occurs where
raccoons are present and frequently follows after
a bite or scratch from a raccoon.
Recovery is slow and relapse frequent.

146

CHAPTER 12

DISEASES OF THE NERVOUS SYSTEM

Nervous System

The brain is the master of all training, the storehouse of all knowledge, and the controller of all body reactions whether voluntary or involuntary. In the hind brain, such automatic reactions as breathing, heart beat, and intestinal motions are controlled. The cerebrum, or forebrain, utilizes stored knowledge to perform tricks, bark, and indulge in any other kind of voluntary action. The Cerebellum coordinates the body, allowing the animal to stand, balance, and run. Various parts of the brain influence reflex actions, glandular control, muscle control and body functions. The spinal cord carries nerves branching out, to the body, channels through which the wishes of the brain are conveyed. Sometimes the spinal cord causes reflex reaction, but it always signals the brain. Throughout the body, there are different receptors which gather stimuli and pass them up the nerves to the brain.

Conditions of nervousness, epilepsy and hysteria are functional disorders of the brain. The brain has a certain capacity for stimuli. If this capacity is exceeded a functional disorder can occur. Normally this does not happen except in conditions such as extreme electrical shock, but the capacity can be lowered by heredity or disease to allow more common occurrences. These are treated with tranquilizers, sedatives and epileptic-treatment-type drugs.

Intercranial hemorrhage and concussion are common occurrences from trauma, usually after auto accidents.

Encephalitis

Encephalitis is an inflammation of the brain substance. It results in nervous disorders such as convulsion, paralysis, chorea (muscle twitches) and blindness.

Distemper is the most common cause but there are non-distemper viruses reported that can also cause encephalitis. Rabies is another virus that affects the brain. Bacterial infection is possible (especially Streptococcus) as well as protozoan (Toxoplasmosis) invasion, and a yeast-like fungus (Cryptococcosis). Encephalitis can also be secondary to general body infection.

Each condition should be treated separately and specifically.

Hydrocephalus

This is a congenital condition of increased cerebrospinal fluid (see pediatrics).

Tumors

Tumors are not uncommon and produce symptoms related to their location in the brain. Most primary tumors are cancerous but there are also metastatic cancers from elsewhere in the body.

Meningitis

Meningitis in dogs is not related etiologically to human meningitis. It is an inflammation of the coverings of the brain and spinal cord. It is most often bacterial from an extension of middle ear infection, or from bacteria brought to it via the blood. It can occur with distemper, but this relationship is rare. It is also caused by special neutropic virus or by toxoplasmosis (protozoan) and cryptococcosis (fungus).

Symptoms are pain, depression and abnormal gait. The head may be held forward or tilted.

Treatment is usually with wide-range antibiotics, with confinement and quiet as auxiliary therapy.

Spinal Cord

The spinal cord can be affected by discs (see muscular-skeletal diseases), distemper virus, abcesses, bacteria and trauma. Treatment is directed at the cause and through removal. Abcesses must be drained, and antibiotics used to fight infection and for treating the general disease. Confinement is helpful to keep the dog from further injury. Sedatives are useful in traumatic cases where depression is not already present.

Coon Hound Paralysis

This is a neuritis of unknown cause. It occurs where raccoons are present and is usually associated with Coon Hounds. It often follows 7 to 14 days after a bite or scratch from a raccoon. The dog becomes progressively paralyzed. The paralysis usually starts with the hind end, but even the voice is affected.

Treatment is directed at good nursing and physiotherapy for atrophying muscles. The course of the disease is usually several weeks to several months. Dogs recover slowly and may relapse. Exercise should be encouraged as soon as possible. Most cases tend to recover but the appearance of the animal is marred.

Toxoplasmosis

Toxoplasmosis is a protozoal disease which is general but usually characterized by nervous changes.

The protozoan invades the nerve cells, muscle cells, liver cells, lung cells and varied other body cells. Transmission is through the placenta from mother to offspring. The disease has been known to affect people in households where dogs are infected, but the method of transmission from dog to human is unknown.

The dog shows loss of appetite, fever, and loss of weight. Coughing, difficult breathing, lack of muscular coordination, irritability, depression, paralysis, and other nervous signs indicate lung and nerve involvement.

It is most commonly seen in young dogs, and where unexplained mortality and sickness occurs in puppies, especially when they are approximately 3 months old, toxoplasmosis could be a distinct possibility. Serological tests are necessary to confirm the diagnosis. Pyrimethamine and sulfadiazine are used for treatment but more research into the disease is needed as the treatment now used is not always successful.

Motion Sickness

Car sickness, or motion sickness, is a common and distasteful problem. It is caused by irritating impulses received in the middle ear and sent to the cerebellum. Motion sickness is characterized by drooling, restlessness, vomiting and occasionally diarrhea.

Most animals tend to overcome the problem with time and exposure to car riding but some do not. Generally speaking it is best not to feed the dog for 6 hours before traveling. Provide the animal with periodic stops and rests about every 2 hours when you are on the road.

There are three types of drugs that will help. Some antihistamines have side reactions that stop motion sickness. These do not depress the dog and, therefore, are excellent for working field trial dogs and dogs on the show circuit.

Tranquilizers and phenobarbital also work but are depressants.

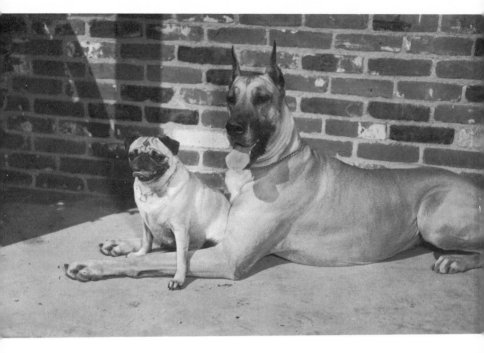

Giantism and acromegaly are associated with
pituitary gland anomalies. Certain breeds are
considered to be normal products of a persistent
pituitary breed change. Great Danes and Irish
Wolfhounds are considered the end result of giantism.

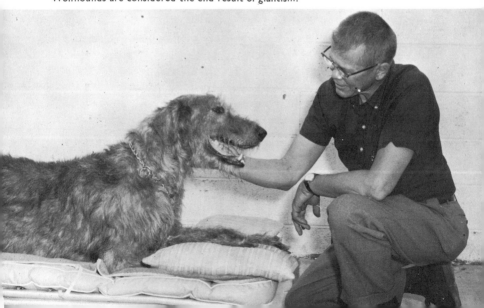

CHAPTER 13

DISEASES OF ENDOCRINE GLANDS

Endocrine glands are ductless glands which add their secretions (hormones) to the bloodstream. The glands which are considered the true endocrine glands are the pituitary, the thyroid, parathyroid and adrenal glands. The thymus and the pineal glands are classified here but are in medical dispute as to whether or not they are true endocrine glands. The testes, ovaries and pancreas are both endocrine and exocrine (ducted) glands.

Pituitary Gland

The pituitary gland acts as a control of the other true glands. It produces a balance so that a high secretion of stimulating hormone from the pituitary, directed at a gland, will cause the gland to secrete. Presence of this secretion from the target gland will cause the pituitary gland to reduce secretion of the stimulating hormone. Therefore damage to the pituitary gland can be at the base of any thyroid, parathyroid or adrenal gland problem.

The pituitary gland also secretes oxytocin which causes contraction of the uterus and milk volume let down. Another of its hormones, vasopressin, has to do with reabsorption of water in the kidney tubules.

Pituitary gland conditions of excess secretion, directly attributed to the pituitary gland alone, are gigantism and acromegaly. While these conditions are rare, certain breeds are considered to be normal products of a persistent pituitary breed change. In this category some authorities consider Great Danes and Irish Wolfhounds to be the result of giantism and Bloodhounds to be acromegalacs. Low pituitary secretion causes dwarfism, extreme emaciation, extreme obesity and diabetes insipidus. The most common defect affecting the pituitary gland and causing increase and decrease changes are tumors, congenital defects, injury, and senile changes. Damage from abcesses or encephalitic infections can also be a primary agent.

Thyroid

Lying in the neck area along the trachea and near the parathyroids is the thyroid gland. While the thyroid gland interacts with the pituitary gland, it also interacts with the amount of iodine stored or available to the body. The hormone secreted, thyroxin, is concerned with regulating metabolism. Hypofunction causes a lowered metabolism while hyperfunction causes an increased metabolism.

Cretinism is a congenital hypofunctional disease present at birth. The cretin is born of a goitrous dam or has a congenital thyroid absence or deficiency. These pups have abnormal coats, enlarged lymph nodes, spleen and thymus, defective calcification and may die early in life. Less severe cases may recover if properly nursed but are often mentally dull.

Some older dogs show poor coats with loss of hair and inactivity which is diagnosed as hypothyroidism. Many tend to respond to thyroid replacement therapy.

Goiter is the most commonly known thyroid disease. It is an enlarged thyroid which clinically may exhibit hypo or hyper thyroidism. It is most common in areas where there is a lower availability of iodine (mid and northwestern USA).

Other conditions such as low vitamin intake, high calcium and dietary imbalance, etc., may interfere with iodine intake thus causing goiter. Treatment is with iodine replacement.

Infections, pituitary disfunctions, tumors and chronic wasting diseases also affect the thyroid.

Parathyroids

The parathyroid gland serves the dog as a calcium/phosphorus regulator. The gland is stimulated by high phosphorus levels to increase blood calcium and calcium absorption. Destruction of the gland causes a drop in blood levels of calcium and a rise in phosphorus. The commonest conditions of the gland are tumor and increased non-tumorous growth due to extraordinary stimulation present in the uremic dog where phosphorus levels rise and calcium levels fall.

Adrenal Glands

The adrenal gland is located near the kidney and has two parts which are unrelated in their production of hormone (the cortex and the medulla).

The medulla secretes adrenalin which acts upon the autonomic nervous system. Adrenalin directly affects the animal, producing stress or fright episodes. The hair rises, the bowels constrict, the blood is channeled to the essential regions, and the heart speeds up.

The dog can live without a medulla but the cortex is essential for life. Steroids are the hormones of the cortex (Cortisone, hydrocortisone, male and female steroids, etc.). The corticosteroids affect the metabolism of water, electrolyte balance, carbohydrate or sugar metabolism, and therefore body energy production, sexual characteristics, and resistance to stress.

Hypercorticoidism will cause feminine qualities to develop in the male, or masculine ones in the bitch. It will also affect the coat and the other functions associated with the cortex. The commonest ailment

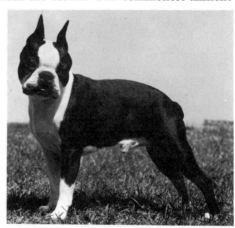

Hypercorticoidism affects the sexual qualities of the animal. Boston Terriers are predisposed to Cushing's disease, the commonest ailment in this category.

in this category is Cushing's Disease. Boston Terriers are most predisposed to this disease at mid-life and beyond. Usually it is caused by a tumor in the cortex. The dog shows a rough coat and abdominal enlargement. The hair drops out to show bilateral patches along the sides and flanks and at functional spots. The animal gradually develops weakness, trembling, and shows an increase in urination and thirst.

Hypocorticoidism may occur suddenly with resulting death in a few hours or days. This terminal phase is usually caused by acute hemorrhagic diseases. The symptoms are vomiting, diarrhea, subnormal temperature, heart failure, low blood pressure, convulsions and death. The condition, in its chronic form, is similar to Addison's disease. The affected animal shows a clinical picture of vomiting, loss of weight, blood changes and pigment changes of the skin. Treatment is with corticosteroids and a low potassium, high carbohydrate diet.

The prolonged use of high doses of corticosteroid can depress the gland, so that sudden withdrawal of cortisone therapy can cause hypocorticoidism and death. Corticosteroid treatment of any great length or amount should be terminated gradually and slowly to give the gland a chance to recoup.

Pineal Body—The pineal body is located in the brain. Its function is unknown and it is not essential for life.

Thymus—The thymus is a gland in the neck and chest regions in young animals. With age it degenerates and disappears. It can become cancerous, and it sometimes causes a toxic condition in puppies (see pediatrics).

Gonads

Hormonal disturbance of the gonads can be local or due to pituitary control. They cause nymphomania without conception in bitches,

Hormonal disturbance of the gonads plays havoc with the dog's reproductive system. The formation of breast tumors is also involved in such disturbances. The bitch in the photo exhibits a well developed breast cancer.

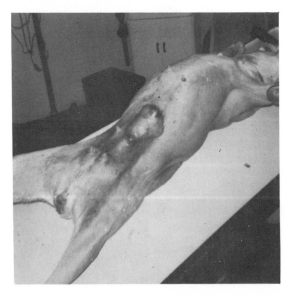

lack of heat periods, general estrus upsets, lack of fertility in both sexes, and sexual changes toward a neuter, or the opposite sex. They also affect associated organs causing uterine and vaginal hyperplasia, prolonged bleeding during estrus, and vaginal prolapse. Hormonal gonad disturbances are also involved in the formation of breast tumors making spaying essential in any canine breast tumor condition.

Diabetes Mellitus (*Sugar Diabetes*)

Diabetes mellitus is a disease of the islets of Langerhans in the pancreas. The islets of Langerhans secrete insulin which regulates carbohydrate/sugar utilization. Approximately .1% of the dog population has diabetes but the disease may go undetected.

The dog exhibits increased thirst, increased urination and loss of weight, while the appetite and food consumption increases. The signs vary in severity, often causing the possibility of diabetes to be overlooked. Laboratory tests will show a high urine sugar and a high blood sugar (normal 100 mg./100 ml. of blood with a 40 mg. variation). If left untreated the dog develops Ketone bodies in the urine due to the upset in fat metabolism and develops acidosis from these acid Ketone bodies. The dog may finally go into a diabetic coma and die.

The objectives of treatment are the same as in human diabetes, through dietary regulation and daily insulin injections if necessary.

The diet should be changed to one of very low fat and lower carbohydrate percentage and higher protein. The insulin dose must be adjusted utilizing urine tests with decreasing doses until a balance is achieved, but continued testing is necessary. Your veterinarian will teach you the principles so that this can be done at home involving only a few minutes of your time daily.

Diabetes Insipidus

Diabetes insipidus is not sugar diabetes but is a failure of the pituitary gland in the brain to produce antidiuretic hormone resulting in a great increase in urination and drinking. There is no sugar increase in either blood or urine.

Administering antidiuretic hormone (*Vasopressin*) will correct the condition and confirm the diagnosis. Daily treatment for the rest of the animal's life is usually necessary.

Eclampsia (*Milk Fever*)

"Milk Fever" usually occurs during the first 3 weeks after

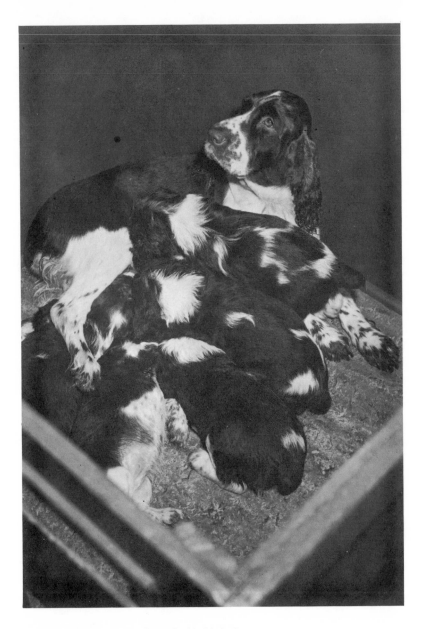

Leaching calcium reserves from the bitch's body
for the production of milk to feed her puppies
results in a lowered calcium content of
the blood and eclampsia, or "milk fever," as
it is commonly called.

whelping. It is caused by a lowered calcium content of the blood due to the lactating bitch depleting the calcium reserves of the body for the production of milk.

The bitch exhibits nervousness and rapid breathing with the first onslaught of eclampsia. Then she begins to stagger, develops muscle spasms and an increased temperature. The bitch eventually becomes "tetnied." These symptoms may occur suddenly or during a 12 hour period.

This is an emergency so do not procrastinate. Contact your veterinarian immediately upon suspecting eclampsia, the cardinal signs again being:

1. *Occurs within 3 weeks of whelping*
2. *Sudden nervousness.*
3. *"Tetanus" like signs.*

When in the final stages treatment is directed at replacing the blood calcium by intravenous injection. The cure is dramatic as usually the dog will be close to normal in approximately 30 minutes. Earlier cases may be treated by corticosteroids. Careful use of corticosteroids on bitches with a past history of eclampsia can help to prevent a recurrence in future lactations.

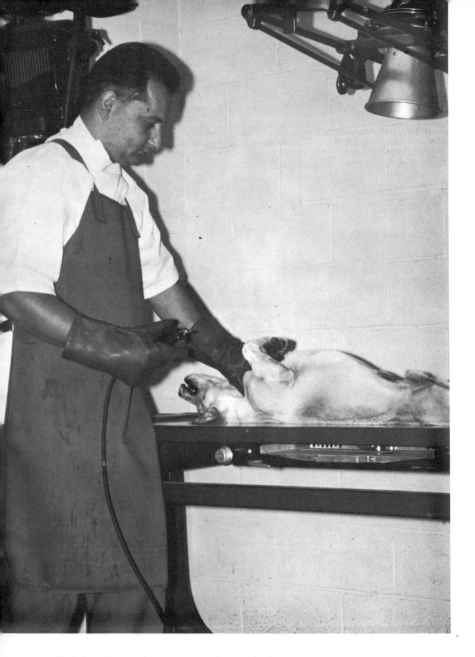

Radiology is not only necessary to diagnose broken
limbs but also is an important diagnostic tool
that allows your veterinarian to
see below the surface. The photo is of the
author and one of his patients.

CHAPTER 14

MUSCULO-SKELETAL DISEASES

Arthritis

Arthritis is an inflammation of the joint. All diseases involving a joint (e.g. hip dysplasia, Legg's Perthes) develop arthritic conditions as an end result.

The joint itself is composed of articular cartilage which covers the opposing parts of the bone, and the synovial membrane which does not cover the cartilage but encloses the rest of the joint and joins the cartilage at its edge. The joint contains synovial fluid which is chemically similar to blood plasma. The articular cartilage, which is nerveless and avascular, is fed by the synovial fluid. The synovial fluid also dissipates heat and, through its phagocytic cells, carries away debris.

The simplest form of arthritis is caused by an increase in joint fluids. The result is a distended joint. If infection intervenes the fluids become fibrinous or purulent. When this occurs erosion of the cartilage and joint pain are common.

If the original cause is not corrected, or unable to be corrected, the condition becomes chronic. Proliferation of the soft tissues lining the joint occurs. This protrudes into the joint and may break away becoming what is known as "joint mice," small, detached bits of cartilage. They become gradually ossified while the articulating cartilage becomes irreparably ulcerated and torn. All this produces pain and restricted movement of use of the area involved. In the extreme case so much new bony tissue may build up that it bridges the two articulating bones and causes ankylosis (bony fusion).

Treatment is instituted via several channels.

a. Treatment of infections, when present, by antibiotics, systemically or locally.

b. Reduction of inflammation by corticosteroids locally or systemically.

c. Reduction of pain through oral administration of aspirin-type compounds.

d. Rest or immobilization.

e. Reduction of weight if animal is overweight.

f. Ultrasonic therapy through deep muscle massage and sound waves.

Congenital Hip Dysplasia

Hip Dysplasia is an inherited condition involving the hip joint. Because of the lack of x-ray facilities in earlier veterinary practices it was not identified until 1935, although the condition had existed for many yeras. It has been identified in almost half of all the A.K.C. registered breeds, especially the large breeds, as well as in cross-breeds.

The basic defect can be one of or a combination of three factors.

1. A shallow acetabulum.

HIP DISPLASIA IN VARIOUS DEGREES

EXCELLENT HIPS

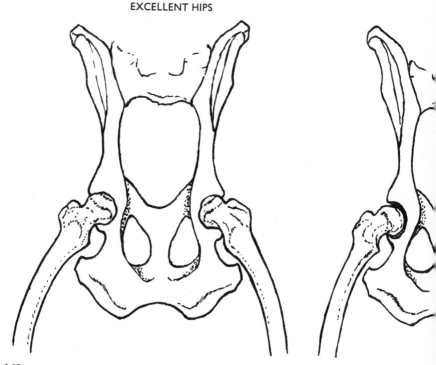

2. *Flattening of the head of the femur.*

3. *Defect in the teres ligament.*

When one of these three conditions exist hip dysplasia is present.

A certain amount of strain will be put upon the hip depending upon the weight and activity of the dog. Gradually the joint will "wear" and arthritis intervene until osteopoetic (bony) material builds up causing an arthritic condition with a specific picture.

Hip dysplasia has been segregated into four grades depending upon the intensity as indicated by the physical x-ray picture, but this physical appearance is also affected by environment and the strain the environment puts upon the affected joints. Regardless of the grade of hip dysplasia the dog exhibits he remains a genetic carrier of the disease and should be eliminated from any earnest breeding program.

There is a similar condition in the elbow (elbow dysplasia) which

SLIGHTLY DISPLASTIC   BADLY DISPLASTIC

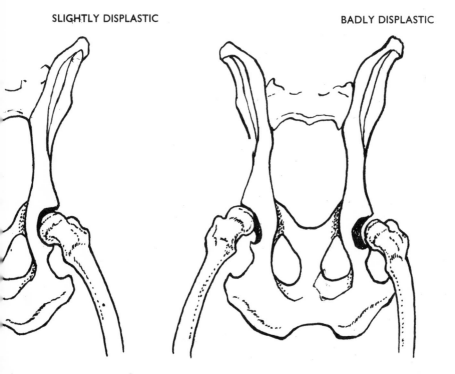

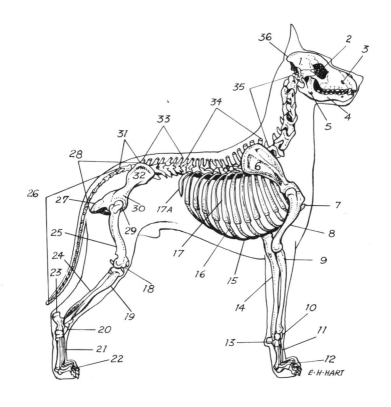

E·H·HART

CANINE SKELETAL STRUCTURE

1. Cranium (skull) 2. Orbital cavity 3. Nasal bone
4. Mandible (jaw bone) 5. Condyle 6. Scapula
(shoulder blade) 7. Prosternum 8. Humerus
(upper arm) 9. Radius (front forearm) 10. Carpus
(pastern joint) 11. Metacarpus (pastern)
12. Phalanges (toes) 13. Pisaform 14. Ulna
15. Sternum (cartilage) 16. Costal cartilage
17. Ribs 17A. Floating rib 18. Patella
19. Tibia 20. Tarsus 21. Metatarsus
22. Phalanges 23. Oscalcic 24. Fibula 25. Femur
26. Coccygeal vertebra 27. Pubis 28. Pelvic bone
entire 29. Head of femur (where hip displasia
occurs) 30. Ischium 31. Sacral vertebra
32. Illium 33. Lumbar vertebra
34. Thoracic vertebra 35. Cervical vertebra
36. Occiput

162

has recently been discovered and which needs much statistical work.

The condition is incurable but the accompanying pain and arthritic changes can be controlled with corticosteroid compounds. Restricted exercise while under treatment, or during "an attack" of pain, is helpful.

An operation for the removal of the head of the femur thus leaving a muscle joint in the area was developed in England for hip dysplasia. It has proved successful for prolonging the useful life of your pet.

Legg's Perthes Disease

This condition is often confused with congenital hip dysplasia but, although the final result is the same, a hip joint with arthritic and osteopoetic changes, the primary lesion is different. Legg's Perthes disease is due to an aseptic death of the head of the femur. This causes wearing and promotes arthritic changes. Thus after the condition has progressed for sometime it is difficult to diagnose whether the resulting degenerated joint is a manifestation of hip dysplasia or Legg's Perthes.

This condition is congenital and has no known cure. Treatment is the same as for hip dysplasia (control of side effects).

Congenital Dislocation of Joints

Toy breeds and breeds where the body structure deviates from the basic normal often have dislocating joints. The knee and the shoulder are most commonly afflicted. Most lightweight dogs can cope with the problem and remain happy, healthy pets. Surgical correction of the knee is possible for the individual, but dogs displaying this anomaly should be eliminated from a breeding program.

Curvature of the Radius

The foreleg of an animal from the elbow to the wrist has two bones: the radius and the ulna. In curvature the radius grows faster, or the ulna has retarded growth, resulting in a radius longer than the ulna and curved compensate, and accompanied by a laterally deviated foot. Correction is surgical.

Uncommon Congenital Deformities

Rudimentary clavicals may be found in the dog. These cause no pathological problems.

Rarely a congenital absence of a rib or part of a rib will occur. Firm membranes in the area usually make the condition of little consequence if it does occur.

Abnormal spinal development with a lack of fusion of the vertebrae is discussed under pediatrics.

Ostrogenesis Imperfecta

This is a congenital condition where the dog is unable to utilize calcium and phosphorus due to a bone cell defect. The result is a slim-boned dog with malformations similar to rickets. The dog may be lame or may have fractures which are almost painless. No treatment is known but Ca/P (calcium-phosphorus) should be adjusted and watched carefully. Many of these animals do not live to adult age.

Osteochondritis Dissecans

This condition occurs in articular surfaces and has been found in the hip joint and the shoulder joint. It is usually the result of trauma and causes a lesion on the femoral or humoral condyle (head). Sometimes a "joint mouse," a small detached piece of bone, occurs. It has been postulated that the single blood vessel supplying the humoral head is insufficient in large breeds thus predisposing them to this condition.

Treatment involves rest and confinement. In order to keep the muscles from degenerating, massage or some type of physiotherapy directed at the muscle with as little joint movement as possible, is often recommended. Intraarticular injections of corticosteroid are often used to relieve inflammation. At times surgery is needed to remove the "joint mouse."

This condition often accompanies "pulled shoulders" in large, or "giant," breeds.

Osteomyelitis

Osteomyelitis is a bacterial infection of the bone. It may be carried to the infected locale via the bloodstream from another area, by extension infection from the surrounding area, from exposure when compound fracture occurs, or during surgery.

Streptococcus, Staphylococcus, and Escherichia coli, are the most common bacterial invaders.

It is necessary in most cases to culture and find the proper antibiotic to stop this infection quickly for, allowed to become firmly seated, it may well become chronic. Surgical scraping, or removal of dead bone, is also often necessary. Any abcess must be drained. Generally speaking the disease should not be taken lightly, but the chance of recovery is good.

164

Mandibular Periostitis

Inflammation of the jaw bones occurs mainly in young dogs and is most common in Scottish and West Highland White Terriers. An atrophy of the jaw muscles occurs accompanied by severe inflammation of the jaws. The cause is unknown but it has been considered congenital. The dog exhibits trouble in eating and the jaws appear thickened. As the condition progresses the mouth is difficult to manipulate and the dog loses weight from lack of nourishment.

Treatment is unknown, but corticosteroids are helpful.

Osteoporosis

This is a metabolic disease where the bone is deossified. It differs from rickets in that rickets is a *lack* of ossification. It occurs in hyperparathyroidism, renal rickets and hyperfunction of the adrenal cortex.

Pulmonary Osteoarthropathy (*Maries disease*)

This is a condition where excess bony deposits occur along the surfaces of the bones, especially the long bones causing an observable thickening. Lameness and difficulty in standing results. Bony deposits also occur in the lung tissue causing a cough or difficulty in breathing. The cause is unknown and no treatment is at present available. The condition is usually terminal.

Scurvy (*Vitamin C deficiency*)

Scurvy is an extremely rare disease affecting dogs as they are generally able to synthesize their own vitamin C. When, for some unknown reason, this synthetization breaks down, scurvy can result. The dog shows bleeding of the gums and skin hemorrhages. Hemorrhages of the bone covering also occur followed by an excess buildup of bone. Treatment is achieved simply by adding vitamin C to the diet.

Renal Rickets

For some obscure reason an alteration of calcium and phosphorus metabolism may occur in conjunction with an abnormality in the kidney. It is thought that, because the kidney lesion results in a lack of retention of calcium and phosphorus during filtration, the body is triggered to mobilize the minerals from the skeleton. An osteoporosis results with all bones affected. Clinically the flat bones, especially the jaw bones, are most affected resulting in a soft "rubber jaw." The parathyroid glands, which have a regulatory effect in bone metabolism, enlarge with constant stimulation. The kidney function becomes progressively worse and calcium deposits may exist in the kidneys, muscles and some other organs.

Clinically the dog shows signs of acidosis (excessive drinking, increased urination, diarrhea and vomiting). The animal is depressed and becomes weak. The breath often has an odor similar to ammonia. Teeth may be loose and the jaw rubbery. Fractures occur easily.

Treatment is directed at the symptoms, especially in relieving the acidosis and thus increasing kidney filtrates and retention of the minerals. Alkaline salt, vitamin C, vitamin D, and calcium must be added to the diet.

Spondylitis

Spondylitis is a progressive arthritic condition of the spinal vertebrae. The dog displays pain upon jumping, may be unwilling to climb stairs, and may even reveal semiparalysis. The onset is usually sudden even though the disease is progressive. X-rays will confirm the diagnosis. Early in the disease the vertebra may grow distinct protruding lips on the lower edges. These may eventually fuse to cause a bridge from vertebra to vertebra. Corticosteroids are used for treatment. After the condition settles down, the dog usually learns to perform normal functions without stress and, therefore, without pain. Surgery may be performed to remove the bridge if the medical approach is not successful.

Elbow Bursitis

This condition is common in large and heavy breeds. The dog reveals a painful swelling on the point of the elbow. These swellings may become as large as an orange on some dogs. The cause is due to injury and bruising of this vulnerable area. Rest and seeing that the dog lies only on soft surfaces, is the only treatment that will bring reduction of the swelling and normal repair after an interval of several months. Injections of long-acting cortisone are helpful, but irritants and surgical intervention are contra-indicated. If the case is left untreated and the lesion becomes chronic or scarred, then surgical removal will have to be resorted to.

Sprains

When your dog has sprained its leg immediate application of cold packs will reduce or prevent hemorrhage or swelling of the area. If it becomes apparent in a few hours that this treatment has not completely eliminated the condition, veterinary help should be sought as torn ligaments or fractures may exist. It may be necessary to resort to x-rays for diagnosis, and immobilization of the limb by splints, casts, etc., for cure.

Disc Disease

Disc disease occurs when a disc lying between the vertebrae ruptures upward causing sudden and often paralyzing injury to the spinal cord. If the disc protrusion occurs slowly and repair or ossification occurs along with it, few or no signs of pain or abnormality may be seen clinically. If the rupture is acute, the dog may be paralyzed or semiparalyzed. Disc ruptures occurring in the neck region are also painful and cause the dog to hold its head back to relieve the pressure. The condition is especially prevalent among Dachshunds and, quite often, Cocker Spaniels.

In some cases treatment is hopeless and the dog is a paraplegic for life. Two methods of treatment are used. Surgical treatment is performed in some cases. This consists of scraping out the offending

When a disc between the vertebrae ruptures upward, the result is called disc disease and is prevalent in Dachshunds.

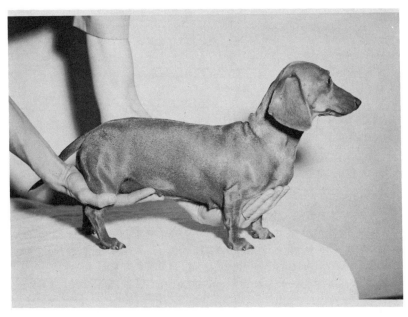

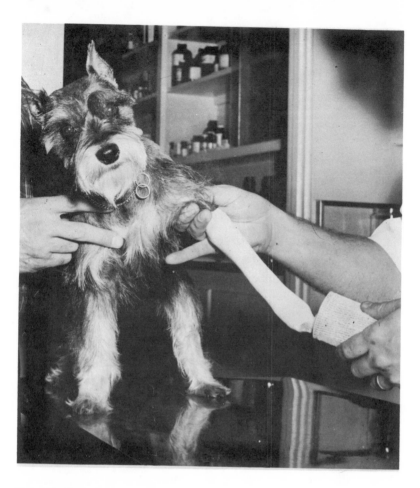

Cast and splints
are common ways of repairing fractured bones.
Internal fixation, the use of pins, etc. may be
necessary, depending upon the severity,
the nature, and the area of the fracture.
Dogs generally heal rapidly when treatment
is immediate and competent.

disc, a procedure especially good in cervical cases and in selected cases where sensation is lacking. In milder cases results are just as good with medical treatment. This involves rest, immobilization, and corticosteroids while the disc repairs. Once recovered there is no guarantee that the condition will not occur with another disc, in fact the dog may be prone to the condition.

Muscular Conditions

Myositis

Inflammation of the muscle may be caused by many things. Trauma, allergy, bacterial and oral infection, poisons (arsenic or lead) and many other causes are involved in non-specific muscle inflammations.

The dog shows lameness, or holds the neck or limb in a peculiar position to relieve pressure, or is unwilling to move. He may have difficulty in getting up after being in a prone position for any length of time.

Aspirin and cortisone compounds are of great help in relieving pain and aiding recovery. Rest, heat and massage of the traumatized areas also are used as nursing procedures. If there is any bone injury resulting in necrosis, the cortisones may be contra-indicated.

Large breeds, especially Great Danes, Irish Wolfhounds, and the tall, fast growing breeds often "pull a shoulder." X-ray should be done if more than a simple muscle injury is suspected as Osteochondritis dissecans may result. If this occurs systemic cortisones should not be used, but rest and often intra-articular cortisones are necessary.

Eosinophilic Myositis

This is a condition of the face muscles that is of unknown origin. The dog shows intermittent attacks where the face muscles swell lending the facial parts a fox-like appearance. The eyes are congested and the lids puffed and swollen. The area Lymph nodes swell and the mouth hangs in a lax, half open position. Eating is difficult for the muscles of the face are painful. The blood count shows an increase of the eosinophils of the white blood cells and eosinophils infiltrate the muscles. As the condition progresses the muscles atrophy and pain disappears, but the jaws lock. The condition is terminal. Cortisone and aspirin are used to reduce swelling and pain.

Muscular Atrophy

This is a shrinking of the muscles usually due to disuse. It occurs as an aftermath of some paralyzing disease (disc, distemper, botulism, etc.). Nerve injury, such as that of the radial nerve where paralysis of the foreleg is permanent, causes atrophy and results in amputation. Injury to the suprascapular nerve is common and results in loss of mobility of the shoulder muscle. Any joint condition will often cause atrophy of the muscles of the affected area.

Wobbles

I use this name to identify a little known condition which has been found in Great Danes. It is of unknown origin. The dog shows a progressive loss of coordination resulting in partial to complete paralysis. I call it wobbles since it resembles clinically a condition found in horses and identified by that name. The condition is usually progressive. Cornell University Veterinary School has seen only approximately six cases. I have seen three cases in my practice up to this time. All these cases have been in young Great Danes and were not related to Stockard's disease (a disease of large breeds involving a lesion in the spinal cord).

Muscular Dystrophy

A myopathy which occurs rarely in dogs is muscular dystrophy. This condition is common in sheep and cattle and is connected with a selenium Vitamin E balance. The muscles affected are pale and flabby and lesions are bilateral. The dog shows weakness in the legs affected. Vitamin E may be used but there is no proof that this has any effect. The condition usually ends in Euthanasia.

Greyhound Cramp

A sudden cramping spasm of the hind leg muscles occurs in Greyhounds while racing. A dog is predisposed to the condition by lack of proper working preparation coupled with cold weather. The symptoms disappear with rest.

CHAPTER 15

FIRST AID AND NURSING

First Aid

Emergencies quite frequently occur which make it necessary for you to care for the dog yourself until veterinary aid is available. Quite often emergency help by the owner can save the dog's life or lessen the chance of permanent injury. A badly injured animal, blinded to all else but abysmal pain, often reverts to the primitive, wanting only to be left alone with his misery. Injured, panic-stricken, not recognizing you, he might attempt to bite when you wish to help him. Under the stress of fright and pain, this reaction is normal in animals. A muzzle can easily be slipped over his foreface, or a piece of bandage or strip of cloth can be fashioned into a muzzle by looping it around the dog's muzzle, crossing it under the jaws, and bringing the two ends around in back of the dog's head and tying them. Snap a leash onto his collar as quickly as possible to prevent him from running away and hiding. If it is necessary to lift him, grasp him by the neck, getting as large a handful of skin as you can, as high up on the neck as possible. Hold tight and he won't be able to turn his head far enough around to bite. Lift him by the hold you have on his neck until he is far enough off the ground to enable you to encircle his body with your other arm and support him or carry him.

Every dog owner should have handy a first-aid kit specifically for the use of his dog. It should contain a thermometer, surgical scissors, rolls of three-inch and six-inch bandage, a roll of one-inch adhesive tape, a package of surgical cotton, a jar of vaseline, enema equipment, bulb syringe, ten c.c. hypodermic syringe, a puppy stomach tube, flea powder, tweezers, ophthalmic ointment, kaopectate, peroxide of hydrogen, merthiolate, a good antiseptic powder, alcohol, ear remedy, aspirin, mineral oil, dressing salve, styptic stick, rubber tube tourniquet, hot water-bottle, tranquilizer or other sedative with veterinary instructions, *your veterinarian's phone number*.

I have prepared two charts for your reference, one covering general first-aid measures and the other a chart of poisons and antidotes. Remember that, in most instances, these are emergency measures, not specific treatments, and are designed to help you in aiding your dog until you can reach your veterinarian.

FIRST-AID CHART

Emergency	Treatment	Remarks
Accidents	Automobile, treat for shock. If gums are white, indicates probable internal injury. Wrap bandage tightly around body until it forms a sheath. Keep very quiet until veterinarian comes.	Call veterinarian immediately.
Bee stings	Give antihistamine cold tablet and use cold cloths over the area.	Call veterinarian for advice.

The photo illustrates the first step in improvising an effective muzzle by using ordinary medical bandage.

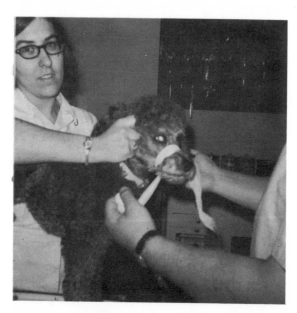

Bites (animal)	Tooth wounds: area should be shaved and antiseptic solution flowed into punctures with eye dropper. Iodine, merthiolate, etc., can be used. If badly bitten or ripped, take dog to your veterinarian for treatment.	If superficial wounds become infected after first aid, consult veterinarian.
Burns	Apply cold water. Dressing with water immersible creams afterward.	Unless burn is very minor, consult veterinarian immediately.
Broken bones	If break involves a limb, fashion splint to keep immobile. If ribs, pelvis, shoulder, or back involved, keep dog from moving until professional help comes.	Call veterinarian immediately.
Choking	If bone, wood, or any foreign object can be seen at back of mouth or throat, remove with fingers. If object can't be removed or is too deeply imbedded or too far back in throat, rush to veterinarian immediately.	

The second step. The bandage is tied behind the animal's head, and he is safe to handle.

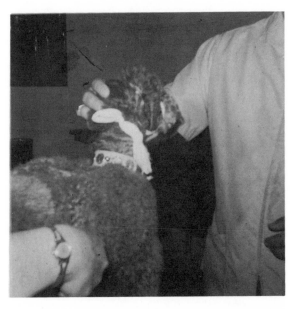

Cuts	Minor cuts: allow dog to lick and cleanse. If not within his reach, clean cut with peroxide, then apply merthiolate. Severe cuts: apply pressure bandage to stop bleeding—a wad of bandage over wound and bandage wrapped tightly over it. Take to veterinarian.	If cut becomes infected or needs suturing, consult veterinarian.
Dislocations	Keep dog quiet and take to veterinarian at once.	
Drowning	Artificial respiration. Lay dog on his side, push with hand on his ribs, release quickly. Repeat every 3 seconds. Treat for shock.	
Electric shock	Artificial respiration. Treat for shock.	Call veterinarian immediately.
Heat stroke	Quickly immerse the dog in cold water until relief is given. Give cold water enema. Or lay dog flat and pour cold water over him, turn electric fan on him, and continue pouring cold water as it evaporates.	Cold towels pressed against abdomen and back of head aid in reducing temp. quickly if quantity of water not available. Call veterinarian immediately.
Porcupine quills	Tie dog up, hold him between knees, and pull all quills out with pliers. Don't forget tongue and inside of mouth.	See veterinarian to remove quills too deeply imbedded.
Shock	Cover dog with blanket. Allow him to rest and soothe with voice and hand. Keep the dog in a quiet and darkened area.	Alcoholic beverages are NOT a stimulant. Bring to veterinarian.
Poisonous snake bite	Cut deep X over fang marks. Drop potassium permanganate into cut. Apply tourniquet above bite if on foot or leg.	Apply first aid only if a veterinarian or a doctor can't be reached.

POISON	HOUSEHOLD ANTIDOTE
ACIDS	Bicarbonate of soda
ALKALIES	Vinegar or lemon juice
(cleansing agents)	
ARSENIC	Epsom salts
HYDROCYANIC ACID	Dextrose or corn syrup
(wild cherry; laurel leaves)	

LEAD	Epsom salts
(paint pigments)	
PHOSPHORUS	Peroxide of hydrogen
(rat poison)	
MERCURY	Eggs and milk
THEOBROMINE	Phenobarbital
(cooking chocolate)	
THALLIUM	Table salt in water
(bug poisons)	
FOOD POISONING	Peroxide of hydrogen, followed by enema
(garbage, etc.)	
STRYCHNINE	Sedatives, Phenobarbital, Nembutal
DDT	Peroxide and enema

Treatment for Poison

The important thing to remember when your dog is poisoned is that prompt action is imperative. Administer an emetic immediately. Mix hydrogen peroxide and water in equal parts or use soapy water. Force eight to ten tablespoonfuls of this mixture down your dog, or up to twelve tablespoonfuls (this dosage for a 50–70 lb. dog, 6 tablespoonfuls for 20–30 lb. dog and 2 or 3 for 5–10 lb. dog). In a few minutes he will regurgitate his stomach contents. Once this has been accomplished call your veterinarian. If you know the source of the poison and the container which it came from is handy, you will find the antidote on the label. Your veterinarian will prescribe specific drugs and advise on their use.

The symptoms of poisoning include trembling, panting, intestinal pain, vomiting, slimy secretion from mouth, convulsions, coma. All these symptoms are also prevalent in other illnesses, but if they appear and investigation leads you to believe that they are the result of poisoning, act with dispatch as described above.

Nursing

Good nursing is an important owner function when your pet becomes ill. Anyone who has raised children will know most of the necessary and basic nursing techniques.

In general if it was not good for the kids it's not good for Fido. Keep sick dogs warm but do not overheat. Blankets under as well as over the dog are excellent. Hot water bottles are very useful but take care not to burn your pet.

Keeping the dog eating is necessary unless otherwise advised by your veterinarian. Broths, bits of meat, baby foods and dairy pro-

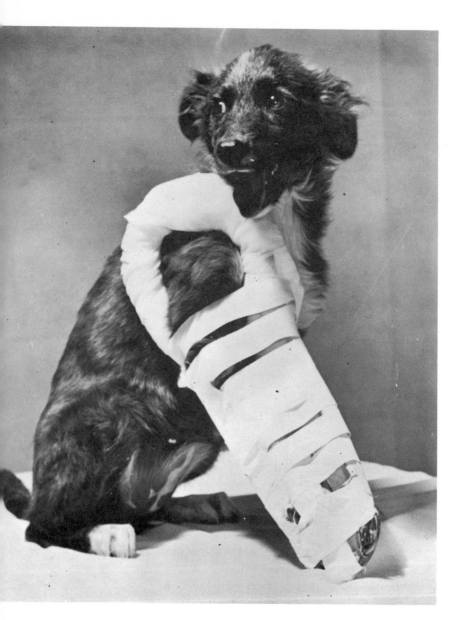

A knowledge of the application of canine
first aid can prove to be of great
importance in an emergency. Without this
vital knowledge one could lose a beloved
companion or an animal of great value.

ducts are very good for sick animals. They are not necessarily any-more nutritious than the normal diet but they are flavorful and bland; two important factors for sick animals. If your dog will not eat he may have to be force fed or fed by intravenous methods in a veterin-ary hospital.

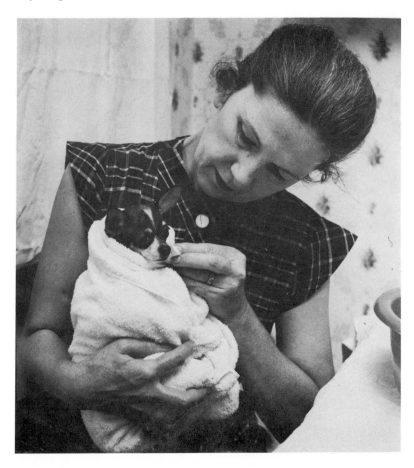

Quiet and rest are as important in recuperation for dogs as they are for humans.

Special dietary changes which may be necessary because of certain diseases and special medications for the canine patient will be given you by your veterinarian. Administering the specific medica-tion will often be your task. Unfortunately threats of no T.V. or

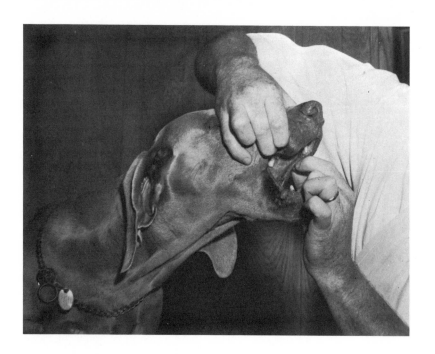

How to give a dog a pill is illustrated in
the above photo.

ice cream will not work with our animals. Unless otherwise advised
giving pills in a small amount of palatable food is the simplest
method and the least distressing to the dog. Many dogs will not take
pills this way, so if your sick pet is recalcitrant you will have to give
him his medicine directly by hand.

The pill should be held in the hand most used by the person (the
writing hand). The muzzle is grasped over the top with the other
hand. Utilizing the lower fingers of the pill hand, the lower jaws are
braced and pressure is put downward while the other hand lifts
upward. The pill is then placed as far back on the tongue as possible.
The mouth is closed quickly, the jaws held together firmly but not
too tightly, and the throat stroked until swallowing occurs. This
latter, wanted event is signaled generally by the emergence of the
tip of the dog's tongue.

Liquids are given at the side of the mouth with the head held
upward. The medication is poured slowly into the pocket at the side
of the mouth, to prevent choking and vomiting.

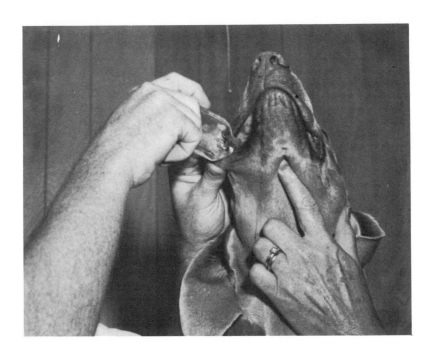

Illustrating the proper method of administering liquid medication.

The rear corner of the lip forms the pocket which is an excellent funnel. Powders are given either as liquid suspensions or in food.

When a dog continually irritates the site of a disease or surgery by licking or biting, an Elizabethan collar will keep him from reaching the area. The simplest form can be fashioned from a plastic bucket. Cut a hole in the bottom large enough to admit the animal's head. Put the head in so that the muzzle points toward the top, then lace the bottom around the dog's collar with a cord.

In order to brace the dog's mouth open while examining the oral cavity a roller bandage can be placed between the upper and lower canine teeth and the animal's mouth held to exert pressure on the bandage to keep him from spitting it out.

When giving an enema at home a common bulb syringe is good but may not be enough. A douching bag or a converted hot water bag is better first aid equipment for this job. Use a soft or pliable tip to keep from injuring the animal.

Bibliography

Archibald, James (editor). CANINE SURGERY Santa Barbara, Cal., American Veterinary Publications Inc., 1965

Benjamin, Maxine M., OUTLINE OF VETERINARY CLINICAL PATHOLOGY, 2nd ed. The Iowa State Press, Ames, Iowa, 1961

Hagen, Wm. A. and Bruner, Dorsey Wm. THE INFECTIOUS DISEASES OF DOMESTIC ANIMALS, 2nd ed. Ithaca, N.Y. Comstock Pub. Ass'n. 1951

Jones, L. Meyer VETERINARY PHARMACOLOGY & THERAPEUTICS, Ames, Iowa. The Iowa State University Press 1957

Kirk, Hamilton INDEX OF DIAGNOSIS, Baltimore Md. The Williams & Wilkins Co. 1939

Kirk, Robert W. CURRENT VETERINARY THERAPY 1966–1967. W. B. Sanders Co. 1966

Kral, Frank and Novak, Benjamin J. VETERINARY DERMATOLOGY, Philadelphia, Pa. J. B. Lippincott Co. 1953

Milks, Howard J. PRACTICAL VETERINARY PHARMACOLOGY, MATERIA MEDICA AND THERAPUTICS, Chicago Ill. Alex Eger Inc. Pub. 1949

Morris, Mark L. NUTRITION AND DIET IN SMALL ANIMAL MEDICINE. Denver Colorado Mark Morris Associates 1960

Pool, W. A. (editor). THE VETERINARY ANNUAL. Bristol, England, John Wright & Sons Ltd. 1960

Rebrassier, R. E. IDENTIFICATION AND LIFE CYCLES OF PARASITES AFFECTING DOMESTIC ANIMALS. Columbus, Ohio. The Ohio State University Press 1942

Runnells, Russell A. ANIMAL PATHOLOGY. Ames, Iowa. The Iowa State College Press 1946

Siegmund, O. H. (editor). THE MERCK VETERINARY MANUAL 2nd ed. Rahway, N.J. Merck & Co. Inc. 1961

Smith, H. A. and Jones, T. C. VETERINARY PATHOLOGY. Philadelphia Pa., Lea & Febiger 1957

Whitney, Leon F. and Whitney, Geo D. THE DISTEMPER COMPLEX. Orange, Conn. Practical Science Pub. Co. 1953

NUTRIENT REQUIREMENTS FOR DOGS. National Research Council 1953

CANINE MEDICINE 2nd ed revised (43 authors). Revised by J. F. Bone 1962

COMPLETE MANUAL OF THERAPY WITH THE METI-STEROIDS. Bloomfield N.J., Shering Co. 1965

INDEX

M

Madura foot 97
malformations 69–74, 139–141, 160–164
mandibular periostitis 165
mange 33–35, 38, 58
Maries disease 165
medicine administration 177–179
meningitis 148
metestrus 111
metritis 111–113, 143
Microsporum canis 35–36
    gypsum 35–36
milk fever 155–157
mites 33–35, 58–59
moniliasis 95
monorchids 69
muscular conditions 149, 157, 164–167, 169–171
muzzling 171–173
Mycobacterium tuberculosis 90
mycotic diseases 94–97, 122, 125
myiasis 30
myositis 145, 169

N

necrosis 169
neoplasms 123, 143
nephritis 107–109
nephroses 109
neuritis 146, 148–149
nocardiosis 95, 145
nymphomania 154

O

obesity 151
osteoarthropathy, pulmonary 165
osteochondritis dissecans 164, 169
osteomyelitis 164
osteoporosis 165
ostrogenesis imperfecta 164
otitis externa 30, 56, 59
otitis media 56–58
Otodectic cynotis 59–59

P

pancreatitis 136–137
papillomatosis 125–126
Paragonimus kellicotti 26
paralysis 147, 149, 166–167, 169
Pasteurella 91
perianal adenoma 45
peritonitis 137
Physaloptera species 26
pituitary conditions 150–151
pleurisy 123
pneumonia 68, 120–122
pneumothorax 123
poison antidotes 174–175
polyps 118
proestrus 111
Proteus 37, 131
Pseudomonas 68
pylonephritis 109
pyloric spasm 130–131
pyoderma 36–38
pyometra 111
pyometritis 40, 115

tumors   45–47, 109, 111, 114, 118–119, 125, 133, 139, 148, 152–155

U

ulcers 143
uremia 109
urinary incontinence 110–111
urolithiasis 110
uterine torsion 115
uveitis 53

V

vaccination 99–105

vaginal conditions 115, 154–155
vomiting   26, 118, 121, 128, 130–131, 133, 136, 149, 153, 154, 166, 175, 178

W

weaning 61–63
Weil's disease 92–94
whipworms 22–23, 131
wobbles 170
worms 17–26, 139, 141, 143